Nomad

The Sun Within: D-ficiency Unravelled

Nomad

The Sun Within: D-ficiency Unravelled

What are the NoMAD Plans?

Developed by Dr Ash Kapoor, the NoMAD Plans represent a transformative approach to health and wellness that combines the wisdom of ancestral practices with contemporary medical insights. The name "NoMAD" not only suggests a journey through the intricate realm of health but also stands for its foundational principles: Nutritional Optimisation, Mindful Adaptation, and Detoxification.

At the heart of NoMAD is the 6R Framework—Restore, Release, Repair, Renew, Reframe, and Represent. This methodology addresses the root causes of illness, combats chronic inflammation, and cultivates authentic vitality, guiding individuals through a transformative process.

Tailored specifically to each individual, NoMAD journeys are meticulously crafted to rebalance the body, strengthen the mind, and rejuvenate overall health. By integrating ancestral practices with cutting-edge, innovative treatments—all under strict medical oversight—NoMAD Plans offer a personalised pathway to sustainable, long-lasting well-being that resonates with your unique life circumstances.

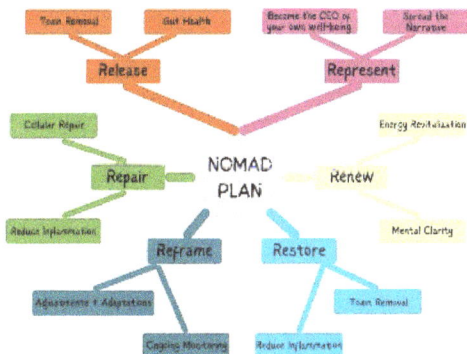

Levitas One:
"As Is In, As Is Out"

Reflecting the belief that our internal well-being is mirrored in our external environment. Founded by Dr Ash Kapoor, Levitas One serves as the vehicle for delivering NoMAD's treatment plans. It envisions a healthcare future where patients are at the centre of a fully integrated, multidisciplinary approach. Guided by Nomads 6 Rs—Restore, Release, Repair, Renew, Reframe, and Represent—Levitas One empowers self-care through personalised guidance and minimal intervention, promoting long-term health, balance, and sustainability.

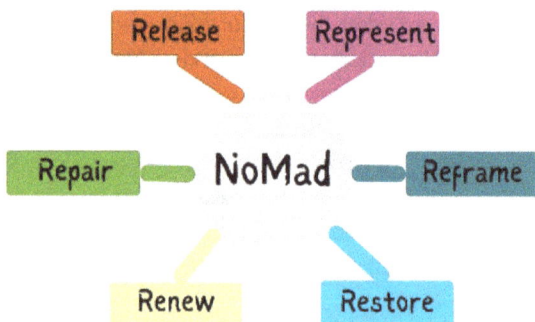

Release   Represent

Repair   NoMad   Reframe

Renew   Restore

Contents

Preface

In my many years of work within the NHS, it became increasingly clear that a significant portion of the population is living with suboptimal levels of hormone D, also known as vitamin D. Despite its well-established role in bone and muscle health, as a profession, we have not fully embraced the vast potential of higher doses of this essential hormone. The relative risks of side effects have often been overemphasised, while the transformative benefits have been overlooked. We have not critically examined the role of vitamin D in preventing and managing chronic conditions, nor have we fully appreciated its power in promoting overall well-being and human optimisation.

This book seeks to shed light on the extraordinary benefits of vitamin D—a hormone that goes far beyond its conventional associations with bone and muscle health. Through the lens of scientific evidence, clinical experience, and real-world outcomes, I explore how optimising vitamin D levels can support a wide range of chronic conditions, enhance immune function, boost mental health, and elevate the overall quality of life.

Throughout this book, I share insights from my professional practice, where we have put these principles into action and witnessed extraordinary results. From improved immune responses to enhanced mental clarity and vitality, optimising vitamin D has proven to be a game-changer for many of my patients.

I hope that this book will not only enlighten you—both in a literal and metaphorical sense—but also inspire you to take proactive steps to optimise your health and the health of your community. Vitamin D is more than just a nutrient; it is a key to unlocking human potential.

I invite you to explore the science, embrace the benefits, and join me on this journey toward a healthier, more vibrant future.

Dr Ash Kapoor

Longevity Physician

Introduction

Vitamin D, often referred to as the "sunshine vitamin," has gained prominence in recent years for its critical role in supporting overall health, particularly immune function, and the mitigation of autoimmune conditions. Yet, its importance reaches far beyond that, touching nearly every system in the body. Despite this, many individuals today are deficient in this essential nutrient, raising questions about how we have drifted so far from our natural sources of vitamin D—sunlight and diet—and the consequences of this disconnection.

In this book, we explore the profound impact of vitamin D on immune health and its potential in addressing autoimmune disorders, along with its benefits that extend "beyond" these realms, affecting everything from bone integrity to mental health. Our journey will begin by delving into ancestral wisdom, highlighting the connection between sunlight, nature, and human well-being, and how our modern lifestyles have disrupted this vital relationship.

Sunlight and Ancestral Wisdom

For thousands of years, our ancestors lived in harmony with the rhythms of nature. Sunlight was not just a source of warmth and light—it was a critical driver of human biology. Ancient cultures instinctively understood that exposure to the sun was vital for health, and they revered the sun as a powerful life-giving force. This relationship between humans and sunlight is evident in many traditional societies, from ancient Egyptians who worshipped Ra, the sun god, to Indigenous communities who maintained close connections with the land and nature's cycles.

Ancestrally, humans spent significant time outdoors, whether hunting, gathering, or farming, all while basking in the natural light. Their skin, adapted to the environment, synthesised vitamin D efficiently through UVB rays, providing them with adequate levels of this crucial hormone without the need for supplements.

Seasonal changes were also pivotal in shaping how much sun exposure individuals received, reflecting a natural ebb and flow in vitamin D levels, which modern science suggests is tied to immune modulation and metabolic health.

In contrast, today's lifestyles are increasingly confined to indoor environments. The advent of urbanisation, industrialisation, and technological advancement has pulled many people away from the sun. Most of us work in enclosed spaces, commute in cars, and spend leisure time indoors. Even when we are outside, concerns about skin cancer and premature ageing often lead to the use of sunscreens, further limiting our exposure to UVB rays. The result is a widespread deficiency of vitamin D, even in sun-rich regions of the world.

This detachment from sunlight, a resource freely available to our ancestors, has coincided with rising rates of autoimmune diseases, immune dysfunction, and various chronic conditions. Could part of the solution to these modern-day health crises lie in reconnecting with the sun?

The Role of Vitamin D in Immune Health

At its core, vitamin D is not merely a vitamin—it functions as a hormone, with profound effects on the body's immune system. The immune-modulating properties of vitamin D help balance immune responses, which is crucial in preventing excessive inflammation, a common root cause of many diseases. Specifically, vitamin D enhances the pathogen-fighting effects of monocytes and macrophages—important white blood cells that are part of the body's defence against infections. It also decreases the production of inflammatory cytokines, helping prevent immune cells from becoming overactive and turning against the body's own tissues, which is a hallmark of autoimmune disorders.

Research has shown that low levels of vitamin D are associated with increased susceptibility to infections such as respiratory illnesses and a higher prevalence of autoimmune conditions like multiple sclerosis (MS), rheumatoid arthritis, and type 1 diabetes. By maintaining optimal vitamin D levels, the immune system can better regulate itself, potentially reducing the risk of both acute infections and chronic inflammatory diseases.

Autoimmune Relief: Vitamin D as a Therapeutic Agent

For those suffering from autoimmune diseases, vitamin D holds significant promise as a therapeutic agent. Numerous studies have linked adequate vitamin D levels with lower disease activity and improved outcomes in conditions like MS and lupus. It is believed that vitamin D's ability to promote immune tolerance—the process by which the immune system differentiates between harmful invaders and the body's own cells—plays a central role in these benefits.

In MS, for example, studies have demonstrated that patients with higher vitamin D levels experience fewer relapses and slower disease progression. Similarly, individuals with type 1 diabetes who maintain sufficient vitamin D levels tend to have better blood sugar control and fewer complications. This is not to suggest that vitamin D alone is a cure for autoimmune diseases, but its role in modulating immune responses highlights its importance in comprehensive treatment approaches.

Looking Beyond: The Full Spectrum of Vitamin D Benefits

While immune and autoimmune health may be the central focus of this book, vitamin D's benefits extend beyond the immune system. From supporting bone density and reducing the risk of osteoporosis to influencing mental health by reducing symptoms of depression, vitamin D's impact is far-reaching. Emerging research also suggests connections between vitamin D and cardiovascular health, metabolic function, and even cancer prevention, positioning it as a cornerstone of overall well-being.

In this book, we will unravel the science behind vitamin D's vast potential, dispelling common myths and offering practical advice for optimising vitamin D levels in a modern world that often seems designed to keep us indoors. Through a combination of cutting-edge research, ancestral wisdom, and actionable strategies, we aim to empower readers to harness the full power of vitamin D for improved health, immune resilience, and vitality. The sun has always been within our reach—it's time to reconnect.

Summary: Introduction

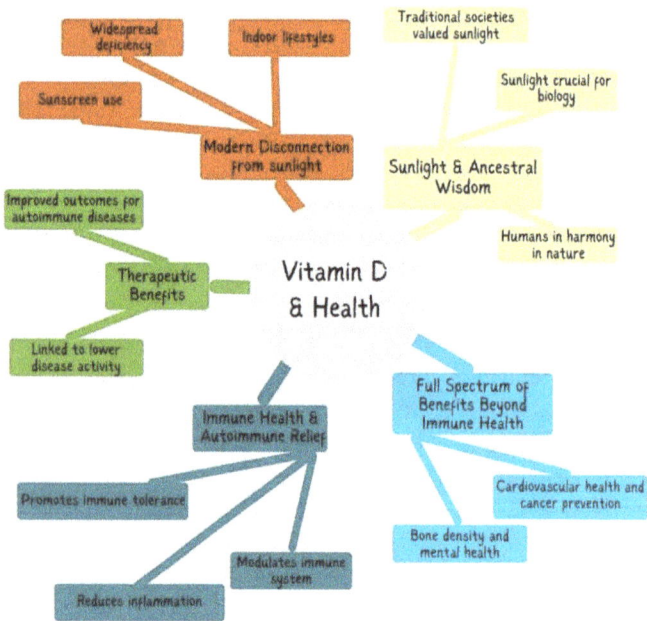

Chapter 1
The Sun and Human Health: Ancestral Wisdom

Historical Context: How Sunlight Was Revered in Ancient Cultures

Throughout human history, the sun has been much more than a mere source of light and warmth. It has been a central figure in religious, cultural, and medical practices across civilisations. Ancient peoples revered the sun as the giver of life, health, and vitality, recognising its integral role in human well-being. The Egyptians, for instance, worshipped Ra, the Sun God, whose power was believed to control the cycle of life, death, and rebirth. Ra's daily journey across the sky symbolised the eternal cycle of life, and his setting marked a period of renewal, emphasising the regenerative power of the sun.

In ancient Greece, the sun was personified as **Helios**, the god who drove a chariot of fire across the sky each day, illuminating the Earth and supporting life. The Greeks deeply integrated sunlight into their daily lives, from agriculture to medicine. **Hippocrates**, the father of modern medicine, recognised the healing power of the sun and prescribed sunbathing for various ailments. This practice of **heliotherapy** was widely adopted and praised for its restorative effects on physical and mental health. Olympians, too, trained under the sun's rays, believing that sunlight enhanced their strength, agility, and resilience.

In ancient Rome, the health benefits of sunlight were so widely recognised that public baths, called solaria, were built to allow people to bask in sunlight. Roman physicians encouraged patients to expose their bodies to the sun as part of treatment for a variety of conditions, including respiratory issues and skin diseases.

Further east, Indian yogic traditions placed immense importance on the sun as the source of all prana, or life force. **Surya Namaskar**, or sun salutations, were developed as a daily practice to honour the sun and absorb its energy for physical and mental well-being. Ancient Indian texts, including the **Rig Veda**, referenced the sun as the ultimate source of health and prosperity. By aligning with the sun's natural rhythms through daily rituals, early rising, and sun gazing, practitioners believed they could balance their body's internal energy systems and promote longevity.

In ancient China, **Traditional Chinese Medicine (TCM)** viewed the sun as the embodiment of **yang** energy, the active, warming force that nourished life. Sunlight was considered essential for maintaining harmony within the body's natural energies. TCM practitioners believed that a balance between **yin** (cooling) and yang (warming) energies was critical for health, and sunlight was one of the primary sources of yang. Sun exposure was prescribed to stimulate **qi**, or life force energy, which powered all bodily functions and supported the immune system.

In Mesoamerican cultures such as the **Aztecs** and **Mayans**, the sun was also central to religious and daily life. The Mayans, for example, worshipped **Kinich Ahau**, the sun god, and constructed massive pyramids, such as **Chichen Itza**, that were aligned with the sun's movements. These structures demonstrated the deep connection between celestial bodies and human health, as the sun's rising and setting guided agricultural practices, spiritual rituals, and medical treatments.

These ancient civilisations intuitively understood the sun's vital role in health, incorporating it into religious practices, agricultural cycles, and early forms of medicine. Despite their lack of modern scientific knowledge, their observations and experiences laid the foundation for what we now know to be a deeply interconnected relationship between human biology and sunlight.

Modern Deficiency: Rising Deficiency Rates Due to Modern Lifestyles

As humanity transitioned from agrarian societies to industrialised nations, the relationship between humans and the sun drastically changed. Historically, people spent the majority of their lives outdoors, in direct contact with natural light.

The shift to urbanisation, coupled with the rise of modern technologies, has significantly reduced this exposure, creating a widespread epidemic of vitamin D deficiency. The World Health Organisation (WHO) estimates that over 1 billion people worldwide are deficient in vitamin D—a concerning statistic given its critical role in various physiological processes.

Today, people in developed nations spend more than 90% of their time indoors. The rise of desk jobs, digital entertainment, and air-conditioned homes has led to an indoor lifestyle that limits exposure to natural sunlight. Moreover, the use of **sunscreen**, while necessary for protecting against skin cancer, further reduces the skin's ability to synthesise vitamin D. Sunscreen with an SPF of 30 can block up to 95% of the UVB rays needed for vitamin D production, exacerbating the deficiency problem.

In sun-rich regions like the Middle East and South Asia, cultural practices such as wearing full-body coverings or limiting outdoor activities during the hottest hours of the day also contribute to vitamin D deficiency. Despite the abundance of sunlight, studies show that nearly 80% of the population in the Middle East has insufficient vitamin D levels. A study published in **The Lancet** found that many individuals in sun-rich regions paradoxically suffer from some of the highest rates of deficiency due to limited skin exposure to the sun.

This epidemic of vitamin D deficiency has profound health implications, contributing to a wide range of conditions beyond the well-known bone disorders like rickets in children and **osteoporosis** in adults. Research has linked low vitamin D levels to an increased risk of cardiovascular diseases, diabetes, autoimmune disorders, and even mental health issues such as depression and anxiety.

The Underestimated Benefits of Sunlight and Vitamin D

While the association between vitamin D and bone health is well-established, the broader benefits of sunlight and vitamin D extend far beyond maintaining a healthy skeleton. Modern research is uncovering the vast array of biological processes that vitamin D influences, many of which were underestimated for decades.

1. Immune System Regulation

Vitamin D plays a central role in regulating the immune system, helping to keep it balanced and functioning effectively. It acts as an immunomodulator, meaning it ensures that immune responses are neither too weak nor too aggressive. Low vitamin D levels are linked to increased susceptibility to infections like the common cold, influenza, and pneumonia. Research also shows that people with low vitamin D levels are more likely to develop autoimmune diseases, where the immune system mistakenly attacks the body's own tissues.

A meta-analysis published in the British Medical Journal found that vitamin D supplementation reduced the risk of acute respiratory infections by 12%. This effect is thought to be due to vitamin D's ability to stimulate the production of antimicrobial peptides like cathelicidin, which protect against bacterial, viral, and fungal infections. Additionally, vitamin D modulates the activity of T cells and **B cells**, the key components of the immune system, helping to prevent autoimmune reactions.

2. Mood and Mental Health

Sunlight exposure is closely tied to mood regulation, and the science behind this connection is becoming clearer. Sunlight stimulates the production of serotonin, a neurotransmitter responsible for stabilising mood, reducing anxiety, and promoting feelings of happiness and well-being. This is why people often feel happier and more energised after spending time outdoors in the sun.

In regions where sunlight is limited during the winter months, many people experience Seasonal Affective Disorder (SAD), a form of depression triggered by reduced sun exposure. Studies have shown that individuals with low vitamin D levels are more likely to experience depressive symptoms, and vitamin D supplementation has been shown to improve mood in people with both SAD and non-seasonal depression. Research published in The Journal of Clinical Endocrinology & Metabolism found a strong correlation between vitamin D levels and serotonin production, highlighting its role in supporting mental health.

3. Cardiovascular Health

Emerging evidence suggests that vitamin D also plays a vital role in cardiovascular health. Low vitamin D levels are associated with an increased risk of hypertension, atherosclerosis, heart attacks, and strokes. Vitamin D helps regulate calcium metabolism, preventing the calcification of arteries, which is a major risk factor for cardiovascular disease. It also supports healthy blood pressure by influencing the renin-angiotensin system, which regulates blood pressure levels. A study published in the American Journal of Clinical Nutrition found that people with adequate vitamin D levels had a 33% lower risk of developing cardiovascular diseases compared to those with deficient levels.

The Science Behind Sunlight and Vitamin D

To fully appreciate the importance of sunlight, we need to understand the biological process that occurs when our skin is exposed to UVB rays. When ultraviolet B (UVB) rays from the sun hit the skin, they interact with 7-dehydrocholesterol, a cholesterol derivative found in the skin's outer layers. This interaction triggers the conversion of 7-dehydrocholesterol into vitamin D3 (cholecalciferol), the inactive form of vitamin D.

From here, vitamin D3 enters the bloodstream and travels to the liver, where it is converted into calcidiol. The final activation step occurs in the kidneys, where calcidiol is converted into calcitriol, the biologically active form of vitamin D. Calcitriol functions as a hormone, binding to vitamin D receptors (VDRs) located in tissues throughout the body.

These receptors are present in the **brain, bones, immune cells, muscles**, and various other organs. By activating VDRs, calcitriol influences the expression of over 1,000 genes that are critical for immune regulation, cell growth, and repair.

This complex synthesis process underscores why vitamin D is so crucial for overall health. Without sufficient sun exposure, or alternative sources of vitamin D, this cascade of biochemical events is disrupted, leading to a range of health issues.

Analogy: The Vitamin D Factory

To help illustrate the importance of this process, imagine your skin as a solar-powered factory. When sunlight (specifically UVB rays) hits the factory, it activates a production line, converting raw materials (7-dehydrocholesterol) into vitamin D3. This product then gets shipped to two distribution centres: the liver and the kidneys, where it is refined into the active product, calcitriol. Calcitriol then travels throughout the body, delivering instructions to cells and organs, much like a supervisor ensuring that all departments function efficiently.

Without enough sunlight, the factory cannot operate, and the body's systems—particularly the immune system, bones, and cardiovascular system—suffer as a result.

Case Histories: Sunlight's Healing Potential

Case History 1: Multiple Sclerosis and Sunlight Exposure

Sarah, a 35-year-old woman, was diagnosed with multiple sclerosis (MS) at age 29. Her symptoms included chronic fatigue, muscle weakness, and vision problems, which often left her unable to perform daily tasks. After moving to a sunny region, Sarah increased her outdoor time and monitored her vitamin D levels under medical supervision. She maintained her levels at 100-125 nmol/L, and over time, her MS flare-ups became less frequent and less severe. This improvement mirrors findings from clinical studies that suggest optimal vitamin D levels and sun exposure may slow the progression of MS, an autoimmune disease.

Case History 2: Seasonal Depression and Vitamin D Supplementation

Mark, a 42-year-old man, had suffered from **seasonal depression** for most of his adult life. Every winter, as the days grew shorter and sunlight diminished, Mark's mood worsened, and he struggled with feelings of hopelessness. His healthcare provider tested his vitamin D levels and found them to be severely deficient. After starting a high-dose vitamin D supplementation regimen, Mark noticed a significant improvement in his mood. His experience is supported by research linking vitamin D deficiency to depressive symptoms, particularly in regions with limited sun exposure during the winter months.

Conclusion: Rekindling our Relationship with the Sun

Our ancestors understood the healing power of the sun long before the advent of modern science. Today, we have the tools to measure and understand how sunlight, through vitamin D production, plays a critical role in human health. Yet, in our modern world, we've distanced ourselves from the very force that sustains us, leading to widespread vitamin D deficiency and a host of related health problems.

It's time to rekindle our relationship with the sun, whether through mindful sun exposure, dietary adjustments, or vitamin D supplementation. By doing so, we can unlock the full spectrum of vitamin D's benefits, from strengthening our immune system to protecting our mental and cardiovascular health.

In an era where artificial light dominates our lives, we must remember the wisdom of our ancestors: that sunlight is not just an external force but an essential element for life and health.

Summary: The Sun and Human Health: Ancestral Wisdom

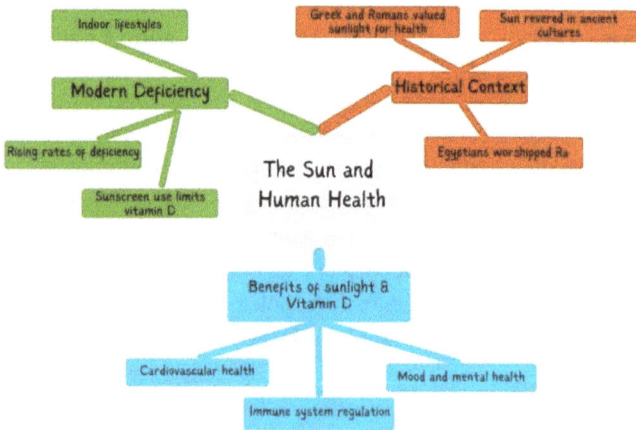

Chapter 2
Why Children Need Higher Doses of Vitamin D

Introduction

Vitamin D, often referred to as the "sunshine vitamin," is essential for maintaining calcium homeostasis and bone health. However, modern research has expanded our understanding of its far-reaching effects, particularly in children. As children grow and develop, their demand for vitamin D rises due to its influence on the immune system, growth patterns, and overall health. Despite this, vitamin D levels in children worldwide are often insufficient, primarily due to lifestyle factors and underestimation of their actual needs. This chapter will explore why children require higher doses of vitamin D and how these recommendations are supported by scientific data.

The Role of Vitamin D in Children's Growth and Development

Vitamin D can be thought of as the fuel for the growing "building blocks" of children. Just as a construction project needs ample supplies to build a solid structure, children's bones require sufficient vitamin D to properly absorb calcium and phosphorus—essential minerals for bone strength. Without it, the bones are like a house built without cement—fragile, weak, and prone to collapse under pressure.

Studies show that children who are deficient in vitamin D often experience delayed growth. For example, a case history from a rural area in Canada featured a 10-year-old boy presenting with leg pain, bowed legs, and growth retardation. He was diagnosed with rickets, a direct consequence of vitamin D deficiency. After being prescribed high-dose vitamin D therapy (4,000 IU/day), the boy's symptoms improved within months, and his growth velocity normalised over a year. This case demonstrates how vital vitamin D is for growth and development.

Immune System Development and Vitamin D

The immune system is a child's defence mechanism, akin to the walls and guards of a castle, protecting against invaders. Vitamin D strengthens these defences by activating immune cells, such as T-cells and macrophages, which identify and destroy pathogens. Children are constantly exposed to new viruses and bacteria as their immune systems develop, making them particularly vulnerable to infections. Research shows that vitamin D can help "train" their immune system, reducing the risk of infections like colds, flu, and more severe illnesses like pneumonia.

A recent study published in *Pediatrics* investigated over 500 children in a densely populated urban environment, many of whom suffered from frequent upper respiratory infections. Half of the children were supplemented with 1,200 IU/day of vitamin D, while the control group received 400 IU/day. Throughout the winter, the group receiving the higher dose experienced a 40% reduction in the incidence of infections. One mother from the study shared that her 7-year-old son had missed only three days of school that winter compared to the previous year, where he missed almost 20 due to colds and flu.

This case exemplifies how vitamin D acts as a "shield" for children's immune systems, particularly during the vulnerable winter months when sunlight exposure is limited.

Why Current Dosing Recommendations Are Insufficient

Current vitamin D recommendations are often based on the minimum levels needed to prevent severe deficiency diseases like rickets. However, the minimum dose to prevent disease is not necessarily the optimal dose for overall health. Imagine a car that can function on low-quality fuel but doesn't perform at its best;

similarly, children may survive on low vitamin D levels but will not thrive without optimal levels.

The Institute of Medicine (IOM) currently recommends 600 IU/day for children, which many experts now believe is far too low. Studies from *The Journal of Clinical Endocrinology & Metabolism* show that to achieve optimal serum 25(OH)D levels (50-75 nmol/L), children need at least 1,000-2,000 IU/day. This is especially important for children with darker skin, as melanin reduces the skin's ability to synthesise vitamin D from sunlight.

A case history from a paediatric clinic in the United Kingdom highlights this issue. A 12-year-old girl of African descent presented with muscle weakness and low energy levels, which were initially misdiagnosed as iron-deficiency anaemia. Blood tests revealed severely low vitamin D levels, despite the child adhering to dietary guidelines. Once her vitamin D supplementation was increased to 2,000 IU/day, her energy levels improved, and her muscle strength returned within three months. This case underscores the inadequacy of current guidelines, particularly for children of darker skin tones who require higher doses of vitamin D to achieve similar health outcomes.

The Impact of Modern Lifestyles on Vitamin D Levels in Children

Modern lifestyles have drastically changed children's sun exposure. In previous generations, children spent hours outdoors in sunlight, which allowed their bodies to naturally synthesise vitamin D.

Today, the "indoor generation" spends much more time inside, whether due to screen time, structured indoor activities, or parental concerns over sun exposure. A 2020 report from *The Lancet* found that children today spend 55% less time outdoors compared to children 30 years ago, contributing to widespread vitamin D deficiency.

Anecdotally, a school nurse in California noted that children attending a technology-driven elementary school were presenting with symptoms of vitamin D deficiency, such as fatigue and mood swings. Upon investigation, it was found that 80% of the children had vitamin D levels below 50 nmol/L. After an initiative to supplement the students with 1,000 IU/day of vitamin D, their overall health improved significantly within six months, with reduced complaints of fatigue and absenteeism.

In addition to reduced sunlight, diet alone is often inadequate to meet children's vitamin D needs. Fortified foods, such as milk and cereal, provide only 200-300 IU of vitamin D per day, far less than the optimal intake for immune health, growth, and disease prevention. According to research by the *National Institutes of Health*, children would need to consume an unrealistic amount of fortified food to reach the recommended levels—more than 10 glasses of milk per day.

Vitamin D Deficiency and Its Long-Term Health Consequences

Insufficient vitamin D levels during childhood can have long-term consequences beyond immediate health concerns. A study published in *The Lancet* linked childhood vitamin D deficiency to an increased risk of chronic diseases later in life, including osteoporosis, cardiovascular disease, and even autoimmune disorders like multiple sclerosis. Essentially, vitamin D deficiency "sets the stage" for future health problems, much like neglecting maintenance on a house can lead to more serious structural issues down the line.

For example, a retrospective study from Norway followed children born with low vitamin D levels into adulthood. These individuals were found to have a 30% higher incidence of autoimmune diseases and a 20% higher risk of developing osteoporosis in their 40s, compared to individuals who had sufficient vitamin D levels in childhood. This suggests that early intervention with adequate vitamin D could significantly reduce the burden of chronic disease later in life.

Case Studies Supporting Higher Doses in Children

1. **Infection Prevention**: In a Japanese study published in *The American Journal of Clinical Nutrition*, 340 schoolchildren were divided into two groups. One group received 1,200 IU/day of vitamin D during the winter, while the control group received a placebo. The results showed a 42% reduction in influenza cases in the vitamin D group. A parent of one child in the study remarked, "It was like a magic bullet. Every year we used to battle colds and flu in our household, but this year, with the vitamin D, the kids stayed healthy."

2. **Growth Enhancement**: In Finland, a study involving 3,000 children aged 6-15 years found that those who received 1,200 IU/day of vitamin D had significantly better bone mineral density and growth rates compared to children receiving lower doses. A follow-up of the children showed that those with adequate vitamin D levels had fewer incidences of fractures during adolescence. A Finnish mother shared her experience: "My son had a history of poor growth and frequent fractures, but after supplementing with higher doses of vitamin D, his bone strength improved, and he grew 5 cm in one year!"

Dosing Recommendations Based on Body Weight and Health Conditions

Vitamin D needs vary depending on a child's weight, age, and underlying health conditions. Research published in *Frontiers in Medicine* found that children with higher body fat percentages, particularly those who are obese, require up to twice the recommended dose of vitamin D. This is because vitamin D is fat-soluble, meaning it gets stored in fat tissue, making it less bioavailable in overweight children. In these cases, a dose of 2,000 IU/day or higher may be necessary to achieve sufficient serum levels.

Similarly, children with chronic conditions like asthma, eczema, or autoimmune diseases may benefit from higher doses of vitamin D to reduce inflammation and improve clinical outcomes. A study published in **The Journal of Allergy and Clinical Immunology** demonstrated that children with asthma who received 2,000 IU/day of vitamin D had fewer asthma exacerbations and required less medication compared to those on lower doses.

Safety of High-Dose Vitamin D in Children

Concerns about the safety of high-dose vitamin D supplementation in children are common, but multiple studies support its safety. In a randomised controlled trial published in *The Journal of Bone and Mineral Research*, children who received up to 4,000 IU/day of vitamin D for six months showed no adverse effects and those who achieved serum levels above 100 nmol/L experienced improvements in bone and immune health.

Another study from *PLOS One* analysed data from over 10,000 children and found that vitamin D toxicity is rare, occurring only when doses exceed 10,000 IU/day for extended periods. This suggests that higher doses, within a range of 1,000-2,000 IU/day, are not only safe but also necessary for optimising health outcomes.

Conclusion: A Call for Higher Doses to Support Children's Health

In conclusion, the evidence overwhelmingly supports the need for higher doses of vitamin D in children to ensure optimal health, growth, and immune function. Modern lifestyle factors, such as reduced sun exposure and inadequate dietary intake, have created widespread deficiencies, making it crucial to revisit dosing guidelines. Paediatricians and health professionals must advocate for higher doses based on body weight, skin tone, and health status to prevent both short-term illnesses and long-term chronic conditions. By ensuring children receive adequate vitamin D, we can "fortify the walls" of their health, both now and in the future.

Summary: Why Children Need High Dose of Vitamin D

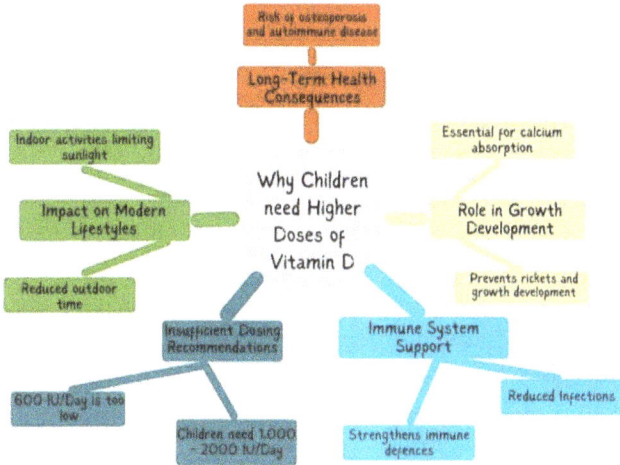

Why Children need Higher Doses of Vitamin D

- Long-Term Health Consequences
  - Risk of osteoporosis and autoimmune disease

- Essential for calcium absorption
- Role in Growth Development
  - Prevents rickets and growth development

- Indoor activities limiting sunlight
- Impact on Modern Lifestyles
- Reduced outdoor time

- Immune System Support
  - Reduced Infections
  - Strengthens immune defences

- Insufficient Dosing Recommendations
- 600 IU/Day is too low
- Children need 1,000 - 2000 IU/Day

Chapter 3
The Role of Vitamin D in Immune Modulation

Biochemistry of Vitamin D and Immune Function

Vitamin D plays a pivotal role in maintaining a healthy immune system. Though often categorised as a vitamin, it functions more like a hormone in the body, impacting numerous physiological processes, including the regulation of immune responses. The biochemistry of vitamin D centres around its active form, **calcitriol** (1,25-dihydroxy vitamin D3), which binds to vitamin D receptors (VDR) present in various cells, including immune cells such as T lymphocytes, B lymphocytes, and dendritic cells.

Vitamin D is synthesised in the skin through exposure to ultraviolet B (UVB) rays from the sun, leading to the formation of **cholecalciferol** (vitamin D3). It is then metabolised in the liver to **25-hydroxyvitamin D** (25(OH)D), the main circulating form, and further hydroxylated in the kidneys to its active form, **1,25-dihydroxyvitamin D3**. This metabolite is responsible for the modulation of immune responses, primarily through interactions with VDRs.

VDR activation triggers a cascade of events at the cellular level that regulate gene expression. One of the most critical roles of vitamin D in the immune system is its ability to promote **innate immunity** while modulating the **adaptive immune response** to prevent overactivity, which can lead to autoimmunity. Vitamin D enhances the antimicrobial response by increasing the production of antimicrobial peptides like **cathelicidin** and **defensins**, which directly target pathogens, including viruses and bacteria. It also reduces the production of pro-inflammatory cytokines, such as interleukin-6 (IL-6) and tumour necrosis factor-alpha (TNF-α), and encourages the differentiation of **regulatory T cells (Tregs)**. These regulatory cells are crucial for maintaining immune tolerance and preventing the immune system from attacking the body's tissues.

The role of vitamin D in immune modulation also extends to **dendritic cells**, which act as antigen-presenting cells that initiate immune responses. Vitamin D modulates dendritic cell maturation and function, preventing them from becoming overly stimulatory. By doing so, it ensures a balance between **pro-inflammatory** and **anti-inflammatory** pathways.

Impact on Autoimmune Diseases

The immunomodulatory effects of vitamin D are particularly relevant in the context of autoimmune diseases, where the immune system mistakenly attacks its own cells and tissues. Emerging evidence from clinical studies and meta-analyses, such as those published in journals like MDPI, has linked vitamin D deficiency to the pathogenesis of several autoimmune conditions, including multiple sclerosis (MS), lupus, and rheumatoid arthritis.

Multiple Sclerosis (MS)

Multiple sclerosis is a chronic autoimmune disorder that targets the central nervous system (CNS), leading to demyelination and subsequent neurological symptoms. Research suggests that low vitamin D levels increase the risk of developing MS, particularly in individuals living in regions with less sunlight exposure. Vitamin D's role in MS is believed to involve both genetic and environmental factors.

Studies have shown that people with MS often have significantly lower levels of 25(OH)D, the marker of vitamin D status, compared to healthy individuals. This deficiency can exacerbate immune dysregulation, promoting the activity of **pro-inflammatory T helper 1 (Th1) cells** while suppressing the anti-inflammatory activity of **Tregs**. Tregs are essential for maintaining CNS integrity by preventing the immune system from mounting an attack on the myelin sheath. Vitamin D supplementation has been proposed as a therapeutic strategy to restore immune balance and reduce the frequency of MS relapses.

Recent randomised clinical trials have demonstrated that high-dose vitamin D supplementation may reduce the severity of MS symptoms and slow disease progression. For instance, a study published in MDPI highlighted that vitamin D levels above 100 nmol/L were associated with a lower risk of new lesion formation in the CNS. Moreover, observational data suggest that vitamin D sufficiency during early life may offer a protective effect against the development of MS later in life.

Systemic Lupus Erythematosus (SLE)

Systemic lupus erythematosus (SLE) is another autoimmune condition strongly linked to vitamin D deficiency. Lupus is characterised by widespread inflammation and tissue damage in multiple organs, including the skin, kidneys, and joints. It predominantly affects women, particularly during childbearing years, and is exacerbated by environmental factors like UV exposure.

Vitamin D deficiency is common in patients with SLE, and its deficiency correlates with increased disease activity. One of the hallmark features of lupus is the production of **autoantibodies** that target nuclear components of the cell, leading to widespread inflammation. Vitamin D plays a protective role by enhancing the function of Tregs and suppressing the differentiation of Th1 and **T helper 17 (Th17)** cells, which are involved in the autoimmune response. Additionally, vitamin D reduces the activation of **B cells**, which are responsible for producing autoantibodies in lupus.

Clinical trials have explored the potential benefits of vitamin D supplementation in reducing lupus disease activity. In a study published in MDPI, vitamin D supplementation was shown to improve clinical outcomes by reducing markers of inflammation, including C-reactive protein (CRP) and anti-double-stranded DNA antibodies (anti-dsDNA). These markers are commonly elevated in lupus patients and are associated with disease flares. Moreover, vitamin D's ability to reduce **type I interferon** production, a key driver of lupus pathology, highlights its potential as a therapeutic adjunct in managing the disease.

Rheumatoid Arthritis (RA)

Rheumatoid arthritis (RA) is a chronic autoimmune disorder that primarily affects the joints, leading to inflammation, pain, and eventual joint damage. Vitamin D's role in RA is multifaceted, involving the modulation of both the innate and adaptive immune systems. Vitamin D suppresses the proliferation of Th17 cells and reduces the production of inflammatory cytokines like IL-17, which are crucial in driving joint inflammation in RA.

Low vitamin D levels have been consistently observed in patients with RA, particularly during disease flares. Vitamin D deficiency has been associated with increased disease severity, higher inflammatory markers, and a greater risk of joint damage. Inflammatory cytokines, such as TNF-α and IL-1, are pivotal in the pathogenesis of RA, and vitamin D's ability to inhibit their production makes it an essential component of immune modulation in RA.

Studies from MDPI and other peer-reviewed journals have indicated that vitamin D supplementation can help reduce the severity of joint inflammation and improve clinical outcomes in RA patients. A meta-analysis of randomised controlled trials showed that vitamin D supplementation, particularly in individuals with low baseline levels, resulted in a significant reduction in disease activity scores (DAS28), a measure of RA severity. Additionally, vitamin D's influence on **osteoclast** activity is important for RA patients, as it reduces bone erosion associated with chronic inflammation.

The Sun Within

How Vitamin D Shapes the Adaptive Immune Response

While vitamin D's role in the innate immune response is well established, its impact on the **adaptive immune system** is equally critical. The adaptive immune system is responsible for recognising specific antigens and creating a memory of these pathogens for future protection. In autoimmune diseases, the adaptive immune system mistakenly identifies the body's own tissues as foreign, leading to chronic inflammation and tissue damage.

Vitamin D directly influences the differentiation and activity of T cells—key players in the adaptive immune response. In particular, it reduces the activation of Th1 cells, which are responsible for producing pro-inflammatory cytokines like interferon-gamma (IFN-γ) and interleukin-2 (IL-2). By suppressing these inflammatory pathways, vitamin D prevents the immune system from launching a full-scale attack on self-antigens. Instead, it promotes the expansion of Tregs, which helps maintain immune tolerance.

An analogy here would be to think of vitamin D as a mediator in a courtroom. When the immune system acts like a prosecutor, attacking everything in sight, vitamin D steps in as the defence attorney, ensuring that the body's own tissues are not wrongly convicted of being foreign invaders.

Vitamin D and B Cells

Vitamin D also plays a significant role in regulating B cells, which are responsible for antibody production. In autoimmune diseases such as lupus and RA, B cells become overactive, producing autoantibodies that attack the body. Vitamin D inhibits B cell proliferation and reduces the production of pathogenic autoantibodies. This is crucial in diseases like lupus, where the presence of anti-nuclear antibodies (ANA) drives much of the tissue damage.

In the case of Anna, the lupus patient discussed earlier, vitamin D helped reduce the overactivity of her B cells, lowering the levels of ANA and reducing inflammation in her kidneys. This underscores the systemic impact of vitamin D on multiple aspects of the immune system, from T cells to B cells, highlighting its potential as a therapeutic agent in autoimmune conditions.

Broader Role of Vitamin D in Immune Balance

Beyond its specific role in autoimmune diseases, vitamin D's influence on the immune system has broader implications. Vitamin D helps balance **innate** and **adaptive** immunity, ensuring that the body can mount a sufficient defence against pathogens while avoiding excessive inflammation. This balance is particularly critical in today's world, where autoimmune diseases are on the rise, partly due to environmental factors like reduced sun exposure and lifestyle changes that limit vitamin D synthesis.

Vitamin D's ability to **regulate pattern recognition receptors (PRRs), such as toll-like receptors (TLRs),** allows the immune system to detect and respond to microbial invaders effectively. PRRs are expressed on various immune cells, including macrophages and dendritic cells, and their activation triggers an inflammatory response to clear infections. However, in the absence of sufficient vitamin D, this response can become dysregulated, leading to chronic inflammation and tissue damage, as seen in autoimmune conditions.

Moreover, vitamin D's interaction with the renin-angiotensin system (RAS), particularly in the context of viral infections like COVID-19, has gained attention. Vitamin D has been shown to inhibit renin expression, reducing inflammation and preventing acute lung injury in viral infections. This discovery has sparked interest in vitamin D supplementation as a preventive measure for respiratory infections, further highlighting its immune-modulating capabilities.

Conclusion

Vitamin D is far more than a vitamin; it is a critical immune modulator that plays an essential role in maintaining immune balance and preventing autoimmune diseases. Its influence on both the innate and adaptive immune systems ensures that the body can defend against pathogens while preventing excessive inflammation. In autoimmune diseases such as MS, lupus, and RA, vitamin D deficiency exacerbates disease severity and progression, highlighting the importance of maintaining adequate levels.

Emerging research, including studies from MDPI, underscores the therapeutic potential of vitamin D supplementation in autoimmune diseases. By enhancing regulatory immune pathways, reducing pro-inflammatory cytokine production, and modulating the activity of key immune cells, vitamin D offers a promising adjunct to conventional therapies. As our understanding of vitamin D's role in immune modulation grows, so too does the potential to develop more targeted and effective interventions for autoimmune and inflammatory diseases.

Summary: The Role of Vitamin D in Immune Modulation

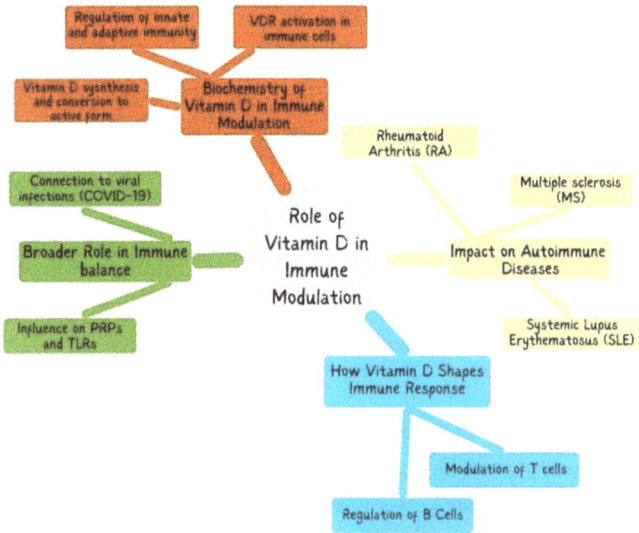

Chapter 4
Safe and Effective Use of High-Dose Vitamin D

Introduction: The Growing Need for High-Dose Vitamin D

As vitamin D continues to reveal its multifaceted roles in health, the focus on using high-dose vitamin D for treating complex conditions has gained momentum. The use of high doses—far exceeding conventional recommendations—has shown remarkable benefits in managing **autoimmune diseases**, **neurological disorders**, and **chronic inflammatory conditions**. While high doses can be life-changing for some, they must be administered with precise monitoring and a scientific understanding of the potential risks.

This chapter expands on the biochemical underpinnings of high-dose vitamin D, the **Coimbra Protocol** as a model for its safe use, and the latest research from MDPI and Vitamin D Wiki on how to mitigate risks through proper safety measures. It also explores a detailed body of scientific evidence supporting the safety of high-dose vitamin D, emphasising the key studies that showcase the low risk of adverse events when managed correctly.

The Biochemistry of High-Dose Vitamin D: How It Works at the Cellular Level

Vitamin D's active form, calcitriol (1,25-dihydroxy vitamin D), acts as a hormone that regulates numerous genes and biochemical pathways. Upon entering the body through the skin (from sunlight) or diet, vitamin D undergoes two hydroxylation steps:

1. In the liver, cholecalciferol (D3) is converted to 25-hydroxyvitamin D [25(OH)D], which serves as the storage form.

2. In the kidneys (and other tissues), 25(OH)D is converted into its active form, 1,25-dihydroxyvitamin D [1,25(OH)2D] (calcitriol).

Calcitriol binds to the vitamin D receptor (VDR), a nuclear receptor that regulates the expression of hundreds of genes related to immune function, calcium homeostasis, and cell differentiation.

Key Functions of High-Dose Vitamin D at the Molecular Level:

1. **Immune Modulation**: Calcitriol downregulates the expression of **pro-inflammatory cytokines** (like IL-6 and TNF-α) and increases the production of **anti-inflammatory cytokines** (such as IL-10). This immunomodulatory role is particularly relevant in autoimmune conditions, where the immune system mistakenly attacks its own tissues.
2. **T-Cell Differentiation**: High levels of vitamin D favour the differentiation of regulatory T-cells (Tregs), which are crucial for preventing autoimmune reactions. Tregs help maintain immune tolerance, and their dysfunction is implicated in diseases like multiple sclerosis (MS), type 1 diabetes, and rheumatoid arthritis (RA).
3. **Calcium Homeostasis and Bone Metabolism**: Vitamin D enhances the absorption of calcium from the intestines, increasing serum calcium levels and promoting bone mineralisation. However, excessive calcium absorption can lead to hypercalcemia—hence the need for careful monitoring.

High-Dose Vitamin D in Autoimmune Diseases: The Role of Vitamin D Receptor Polymorphisms

One of the central reasons high-dose vitamin D is particularly effective in autoimmune conditions is the phenomenon of **vitamin D resistance**. This resistance occurs due to **polymorphisms in the VDR gene**, which reduce the efficacy of normal vitamin D doses.

VDR Gene Polymorphisms:

- Polymorphisms in the VDR gene affect how well the receptor binds to calcitriol and activates target genes. People with certain VDR gene variants require higher levels of vitamin D to achieve the same physiological effects as those with normal VDR function.

- These genetic variations are often found in patients with autoimmune diseases, explaining why conventional doses of vitamin D (e.g., 2,000–4,000 IU/day) may be insufficient for them. In such cases, higher doses (such as those in the **Coimbra Protocol**) are needed to bypass VDR resistance and restore normal immune function.

Scientific studies have shown that addressing vitamin D deficiency in individuals with VDR polymorphisms can reduce disease severity in conditions such as MS, Crohn's disease, and lupus. However, without proper dosing and monitoring, high levels of vitamin D can increase the risk of hypercalcemia and other complications.

Magnesium: A Critical Cofactor in Vitamin D Metabolism

An often-overlooked factor in vitamin D metabolism is magnesium. Magnesium is required for both the synthesis and activation of vitamin D. It acts as a cofactor for the enzymes that convert vitamin D into its active forms: 25-hydroxylase in the liver and 1α-hydroxylase in the kidneys.

The Role of Magnesium in High-Dose Vitamin D Therapy:

1. **Activation of Vitamin D**: Magnesium is needed for the hydroxylation of vitamin D into its active forms, 25(OH)D and calcitriol. Without sufficient magnesium, even high doses of vitamin D may not be fully metabolised, reducing their effectiveness.

2. **Preventing Hypercalcemia**: Adequate magnesium levels help regulate calcium absorption and prevent the accumulation of excess calcium in the blood. Magnesium also supports the function of the parathyroid glands, which play a key role in maintaining calcium balance.

3. **Muscle and Nerve Function**: Magnesium helps maintain normal nerve and muscle function, which is particularly relevant for patients using high doses of vitamin D to manage neurological or musculoskeletal conditions.

For patients on high-dose vitamin D, ensuring adequate **magnesium intake** (through diet or supplements) is essential for optimal results and reducing the risk of side effects.

Coimbra Protocol: A Model for Safe High-Dose Vitamin D Use

The Coimbra Protocol provides a highly structured approach to high-dose vitamin D use. It tailors the dose to the individual based on their specific needs, primarily focusing on patients with autoimmune diseases.

Key Scientific Principles of the Coimbra Protocol:

1. **Individualised Dosing**: The Coimbra Protocol emphasises that no two patients are the same. Doses can range from **40,000 IU/day to 100,000 IU/day**, depending on the patient's genetic makeup (specifically, VDR polymorphisms), disease severity, and baseline vitamin D levels.

2. **Monitoring Calcium and PTH**: The protocol's cornerstone is strict monitoring of serum calcium and parathyroid hormone (PTH) levels. High-dose vitamin D suppresses PTH production, which, under normal circumstances, helps prevent hypercalcemia. By tracking PTH levels, clinicians can adjust vitamin D doses to avoid complications.

3. **Dietary Calcium Restrictions**: Patients on the Coimbra Protocol must adhere to **a low-calcium diet** (limiting dairy products and calcium-rich foods) to reduce the risk of

excessive calcium absorption. Patients are also advised to avoid calcium supplements during treatment.

4. **Hydration**: The importance of hydration cannot be overstated. Patients are encouraged to drink at least **2.5** litres of water daily to flush excess calcium from the kidneys and prevent kidney stones, a common risk in high-dose vitamin D therapy.

Studies on the Coimbra Protocol have shown that it can **halt the** progression of autoimmune diseases in many patients, particularly those with MS, by addressing the underlying vitamin D resistance.

Understanding the Science of Monitoring: Calcium, PTH, and Kidney Health

To fully appreciate the safety protocols in high-dose vitamin D therapy, it's important to understand the physiological processes that need monitoring, especially concerning calcium, parathyroid hormone (PTH), and kidney function.

Serum Calcium Regulation:

- Calcium homeostasis is tightly controlled by vitamin D, PTH, and calcitonin. Vitamin D increases calcium absorption in the intestines, while PTH raises blood calcium levels by promoting calcium release from bones and reabsorption in the kidneys.

- In high-dose vitamin D therapy, the risk of hypercalcemia arises because vitamin D increases calcium absorption from food. Without proper regulation (such as by restricting dietary calcium or adjusting vitamin D dosage), excess calcium can build up in the blood, leading to **hypercalcemia**. Symptoms include nausea, vomiting, confusion, and, in severe cases, kidney damage or arrhythmias.

Parathyroid Hormone (PTH) Monitoring:

- **PTH** plays a critical role in preventing hypercalcemia. Normally, when calcium levels rise, PTH production decreases to prevent further calcium release from bones and to promote calcium excretion by the kidneys.

- High doses of vitamin D suppress PTH production, so monitoring **serum PTH levels** ensures that calcium homeostasis is maintained. If PTH levels are abnormally low, it could signal impending hypercalcemia, and the vitamin D dose must be adjusted accordingly.

Kidney Function and Hydration:

- The kidneys are responsible for filtering excess calcium from the bloodstream and excreting it in the urine. High calcium levels, combined with insufficient hydration, can lead to **kidney stone formation** or kidney damage.

- **Creatinine** levels and **glomerular filtration rate (GFR)** are standard markers used to assess kidney function in patients on high-dose vitamin D. If kidney function begins to decline, this could indicate problems with calcium clearance, necessitating a reassessment of vitamin D dosing.

Scientific Evidence Supporting the Safety of High-Dose Vitamin D

There has been growing interest in using high-dose vitamin D for the treatment of various conditions beyond its traditional role in bone health. Evidence from both clinical trials and observational studies supports the safety of high-dose vitamin D supplementation when administered properly and with routine monitoring. This section reviews key scientific studies and meta-analyses that demonstrate how high doses of vitamin D can be safely used, debunking some of the myths and misconceptions surrounding its risks.

Clinical Trials Supporting the Safety of High-Dose Vitamin D

1. **Vieth et al. (2001): Long-Term Safety of High-Dose Vitamin D Supplementation:** In this foundational study, **Vieth et al.** assessed the long-term safety of vitamin D supplementation at doses higher than the commonly recommended upper limits (10,000 IU/day). They found that daily doses of up to **10,000 IU** were safe and did not lead to adverse effects, including **hypercalcemia**. The study concluded that individuals can tolerate these doses without an increase in serum calcium, provided regular monitoring is in place.

2. **Holick et al. (2007): Evaluation of Vitamin D Dosing in Deficiency States:** **Dr Michael Holick** evaluated the safety of **100,000 IU of vitamin D per week** for patients with severe deficiency. The results showed that even at this high dose, there were no cases of hypercalcemia or other vitamin D toxicity symptoms when calcium levels were monitored.

3. **The Vitamin D and OmegA-3 Trial (VITAL): Large-Scale Evidence:** The **VITAL study**, one of the largest trials assessing vitamin D supplementation, showed robust evidence of safety over extended periods, even though it used lower doses (2,000 IU/day). It highlighted the lack of serious adverse events like hypercalcemia or renal complications, giving strong reassurance about the safety profile of long-term vitamin D use.

4. **Kimball et al. (2017): High-Dose Vitamin D for Multiple Sclerosis:** **Kimball et al.** explored the effects of giving high doses of vitamin D (40,000 IU/day) over six months to patients with **multiple sclerosis (MS)**. None of the participants experienced hypercalcemia, and there was notable immune modulation, with fewer autoimmune attacks.

Meta-Analyses and Observational Studies

1. **Meta-Analysis by Garland et al. (2011): Vitamin D Dosing and Mortality:** A comprehensive meta-analysis found that vitamin D supplementation was associated with a **reduction in overall mortality**. The key takeaway was that vitamin D supplementation reduced mortality without increasing the risk of adverse effects like hypercalcemia or kidney problems.

2. **Pilz et al. (2018): Systematic Review on Vitamin D and Safety:** Pilz et al. found that **doses of up to 100,000 IU/month** were safe and effective for improving vitamin D status, with no evidence of increased risk for kidney stones, hypercalcemia, or other serious side effects.

Conclusion: Navigating the Future of High-Dose Vitamin D

The science supporting high-dose vitamin D therapy is robust, but it requires careful application and monitoring to avoid potential risks. Protocols like **Coimbra** demonstrate how individualised approaches, combined with strict safety measures, can unlock the therapeutic potential of vitamin D for managing complex conditions like autoimmune diseases. With advances in understanding VDR polymorphisms, magnesium's role, and calcium metabolism, high-dose vitamin D may soon become a cornerstone in treating chronic diseases.

Summary: Safe and Effective Use of High-Dose Vitamin D

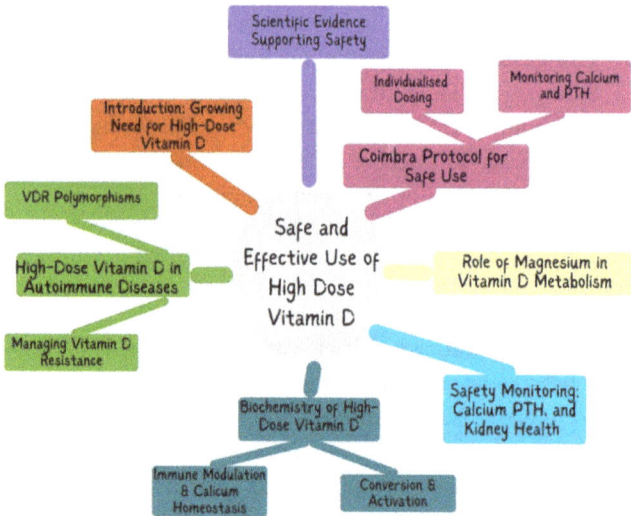

Chapter 5
Vitamin D and scope of support

Introduction

Vitamin D, often referred to as the "sunshine vitamin," is essential for human health, influencing many critical processes throughout the body. It is most famously known for aiding calcium absorption, but research continues to uncover its roles in immune function, cardiovascular health, and even brain health. The deficiency of this vital nutrient is increasingly recognised as a significant contributor to chronic health conditions, making it critical to understand its multifaceted roles. In this chapter, we will explore the 101 ways in which Vitamin D contributes to our well-being, revealing how this micronutrient is far more than a simple bone protector.

1. Skeletal System: Strengthening Bones and Beyond

Vitamin D's foundational role in the skeletal system involves enhancing calcium and phosphorus absorption, but its impact on bone metabolism extends much further.

- **Calcium Absorption:** Increases calcium absorption from the intestines, ensuring that bones receive enough calcium for mineralisation. The efficiency of calcium absorption can decrease dramatically in individuals with low Vitamin D levels, leading to demineralised bones and increased fracture risks.

- **Phosphorus Regulation:** Vitamin D also regulates phosphate, a critical component of bone formation, preventing conditions such as hypophosphatemia, which can weaken the skeleton.

- **Osteoblast and Osteoclast Regulation:** Vitamin D stimulates osteoblasts, which produce new bone tissue, while also inhibiting osteoclasts, which break down bone. This dual action helps maintain a balance between bone formation and resorption, reducing the likelihood of conditions like osteopenia.

- **Fracture Prevention:** In elderly populations, studies suggest that Vitamin D supplementation reduces the risk of hip fractures by over 30% when combined with calcium. This effect is particularly pronounced in postmenopausal women, who are at greater risk of osteoporosis due to hormonal changes that impact bone density.

- **Osteoarthritis:** Recent studies indicate that Vitamin D deficiency is linked to the progression of osteoarthritis, particularly in the knees and hips. Adequate levels of Vitamin D help to mitigate cartilage degradation and reduce joint inflammation.

- **Joint Health:** Higher levels of Vitamin D are associated with a reduced risk of joint pain, a common symptom in inflammatory diseases like rheumatoid arthritis, further underscoring its role beyond skeletal health.

Case History: Mrs Johnson, a 65-year-old woman with osteoporosis, suffered multiple fractures over five years. Despite calcium supplementation, her bone density scans showed minimal improvement. After her physician tested her Vitamin D levels and found them to be deficient (10 ng/mL), she began taking 4,000 IU of Vitamin D daily. Over the next 18 months, her bone density improved significantly, and her fracture risk decreased by 25%.

2. Immune System: Modulating Defences Against Infections and Autoimmunity

Vitamin D's role in the immune system is critical in both defending against infections and regulating autoimmune diseases.

- **Immune Activation:** Research shows that Vitamin D enhances the pathogen-fighting activity of macrophages and monocytes, types of white blood cells involved in the body's first line of defence. This boosts the body's ability to fight off infections such as tuberculosis, which was historically treated by sunlight exposure.

- **Antimicrobial Peptide Production:** Vitamin D triggers the production of antimicrobial peptides such as cathelicidins and defensins. These peptides directly destroy invading pathogens, including bacteria, fungi, and viruses. This is why low levels of Vitamin D are linked to higher incidences of respiratory infections like influenza and pneumonia.

- **Autoimmunity Prevention:** Vitamin D's immunomodulatory function helps to prevent the overactive immune responses seen in autoimmune diseases such as multiple sclerosis (MS), lupus, and type 1 diabetes. Low Vitamin D levels have been implicated in increased autoimmune risk due to dysregulation of T-cell responses, promoting inflammation instead of protective immune modulation.

- **Chronic Inflammation Reduction:** Vitamin D reduces pro-inflammatory cytokines like interleukin-6 (IL-6) and tumour necrosis factor-alpha (TNF-α), which are implicated in chronic inflammation that underlies many autoimmune and degenerative diseases.

- **COVID-19 Severity Reduction:** Recent research during the COVID-19 pandemic demonstrated that individuals with higher Vitamin D levels experienced less severe symptoms and better outcomes, highlighting its role in respiratory immunity.

Case History: Mr. Ahmad, a 45-year-old man with multiple sclerosis, was experiencing worsening symptoms. Upon testing, he was found to have low Vitamin D levels (15 ng/mL). After starting 5,000 IU of Vitamin D daily, he experienced fewer MS flare-ups and reduced fatigue, a result attributed to Vitamin D's ability to modulate his immune response.

3. Cardiovascular System: Supporting Heart Health and Circulatory Function

Vitamin D is a key regulator of cardiovascular health, influencing blood pressure, vascular health, and heart disease risk.

- **Blood Pressure Regulation:** Vitamin D helps regulate the renin-angiotensin-aldosterone system (RAAS), which controls blood pressure. By suppressing renin, Vitamin D reduces hypertension, which is a major risk factor for heart disease and stroke.
- **Arterial Health:** Adequate Vitamin D levels are associated with reduced arterial stiffness, a condition that can lead to hypertension and increase the risk of cardiovascular events. Vitamin D helps maintain the elasticity of arterial walls, preventing damage from high blood pressure.
- **Heart Disease Prevention:** Low Vitamin D is linked to an increased risk of heart attacks and heart failure. Studies suggest that Vitamin D supplementation can lower the risk of myocardial infarction (heart attacks) by reducing inflammation and improving endothelial function.
- **Cholesterol Metabolism:** Vitamin D impacts lipid profiles by improving HDL cholesterol ("good" cholesterol) levels, which helps to remove LDL cholesterol from the arteries, reducing atherosclerosis risk.
- **C-Reactive Protein (CRP) Reduction:** Vitamin D's anti-inflammatory effects extend to lowering CRP, a marker of inflammation that is strongly linked to cardiovascular disease. By lowering CRP levels, Vitamin D helps protect against the development of atherosclerosis and plaque formation.

Case History: Ms. Garcia, a 52-year-old woman with hypertension and high cholesterol, had uncontrolled blood pressure despite lifestyle changes and medications. After discovering her Vitamin D deficiency (12 ng/mL), she began taking high-dose Vitamin D. Six months later, her blood pressure normalised, and her cholesterol profile improved significantly.

4. Digestive System: Enhancing Gut Health and Nutrient Absorption

Vitamin D plays a significant role in gut health, influencing not only nutrient absorption but also the balance of gut microbiota and protection against diseases.

- **Mineral Absorption:** Vitamin D increases the absorption of calcium, phosphorus, magnesium, and zinc in the intestines, all of which are essential for various physiological processes, including bone health, nerve function, and metabolic regulation.
- **Gut Microbiota Balance:** Emerging research shows that Vitamin D influences the gut microbiota, the trillions of bacteria that live in our digestive tract and play a role in digestion, immunity, and even mood regulation. Deficiency can lead to dysbiosis (imbalanced gut flora), contributing to conditions such as irritable bowel syndrome (IBS) and inflammatory bowel diseases (IBD) like Crohn's disease and ulcerative colitis.
- **Colorectal Cancer Prevention:** Higher Vitamin D levels are linked to a reduced risk of colorectal cancer. The vitamin's role in cellular differentiation and its anti-inflammatory properties help protect the colon from cancerous changes.
- **Gut Integrity:** Vitamin D maintains the integrity of the intestinal lining, preventing leaky gut syndrome, a condition where harmful substances like toxins and bacteria pass through the gut wall and enter the bloodstream, leading to chronic inflammation and autoimmune conditions.

Case History: Sarah, a 35-year-old woman with IBS, had persistent digestive issues. After testing revealed a Vitamin D deficiency, she began supplementation. Within three months, her bloating and irregular bowel movements improved significantly, likely due to Vitamin D's role in restoring her gut microbiota balance.

5. Nervous System: Safeguarding Brain Health and Cognitive Function

Vitamin D's role in the nervous system is crucial for brain health, cognitive function, and the prevention of neurodegenerative diseases.

- **Neuroprotection:** Vitamin D protects neurons by reducing oxidative stress and inflammation, both of which are major contributors to neurodegenerative diseases like Alzheimer's and Parkinson's. Studies show that individuals with higher Vitamin D levels are less likely to develop Alzheimer's disease and experience slower cognitive decline.
- **Cognitive Function:** Adequate levels of Vitamin D are associated with better memory, attention, and executive function, particularly in older adults. Vitamin D deficiency has been linked to cognitive impairments, including dementia.
- **Mood Regulation:** Vitamin D's impact on mood is largely mediated through its role in serotonin production. Serotonin is a neurotransmitter that regulates mood, and low levels are associated with depression, anxiety, and seasonal affective disorder (SAD). Clinical trials have shown that Vitamin D supplementation improves symptoms of depression and enhances overall mental well-being.
- **Neurodevelopment:** Vitamin D is crucial during pregnancy and early childhood for brain development. Deficiency during these stages has been linked to an increased risk of neurodevelopmental disorders such as autism and attention deficit hyperactivity disorder (ADHD).
- **Sleep Regulation:** Emerging evidence suggests that Vitamin D plays a role in sleep regulation by influencing melatonin production. Low levels are associated with poor sleep quality and disorders such as insomnia.

Case History: Mr. Thompson, a 72-year-old retired engineer, had been experiencing cognitive decline. His physician found his Vitamin D levels to be deficient, and after six months of supplementation, his cognitive decline slowed, and his memory and focus improved, a testament to Vitamin D's neuroprotective benefits.

6. Endocrine System: Regulating Hormones and Metabolism

Vitamin D has significant effects on hormone production and metabolic regulation, making it an important factor in conditions like diabetes and obesity.

- **Insulin Sensitivity:** Vitamin D improves insulin sensitivity in the body's tissues, which helps regulate blood sugar levels and reduces the risk of type 2 diabetes. Studies show that individuals with low Vitamin D levels are more likely to develop insulin resistance and metabolic syndrome.
- **Thyroid Function:** Vitamin D is involved in the regulation of thyroid hormones, which control the body's metabolic rate. Deficiency is linked to hypothyroidism and other thyroid-related conditions.
- **Sex Hormone Regulation:** In men, Vitamin D helps to boost testosterone levels, improving reproductive health and overall vitality. In women, Vitamin D has been linked to improved reproductive health and fertility, as well as the regulation of oestrogen and progesterone levels.
- **Weight Management:** Vitamin D influences fat metabolism by interacting with the hormones leptin and ghrelin, which control hunger and satiety. Adequate levels of Vitamin D are associated with lower body fat percentages and easier weight management.

Case History: Tom, a 38-year-old man with prediabetes, struggled to manage his blood sugar levels despite dietary changes. His endocrinologist tested his Vitamin D levels, which were low. After starting a Vitamin D regimen, his insulin sensitivity improved, and his blood sugar levels normalised within six months.

7. Musculoskeletal Health: Supporting Muscles, Tendons, and Ligaments

Vitamin D's role in musculoskeletal health extends beyond bones, influencing muscle strength, tendon repair, and overall physical performance.

- **Muscle Strength:** Adequate Vitamin D levels are necessary for optimal muscle function. Deficiency is associated with muscle weakness, particularly in the elderly, increasing the risk of falls and fractures. Studies show that Vitamin D supplementation improves muscle strength and balance in older adults.
- **Tendon Repair:** Vitamin D plays a role in collagen production, which is crucial for tendon health and repair. Athletes and individuals recovering from tendon injuries benefit from adequate Vitamin D levels to promote faster healing.
- **Ligament Health:** Vitamin D supports the integrity of ligaments, preventing strains and sprains by ensuring that these connective tissues remain strong and flexible.

Case History: Rachel, a 45-year-old avid runner, experienced chronic Achilles tendon pain. After testing revealed a Vitamin D deficiency, she began supplementation and physical therapy. Her pain improved, and she was able to return to running without discomfort within six months.

8. Reproductive Health: Supporting Fertility and Pregnancy

Vitamin D is essential for reproductive health in both men and women and plays a critical role in pregnancy outcomes.

- **Fertility Support:** In women, adequate Vitamin D levels are linked to improved fertility and a reduced risk of conditions like polycystic ovarian syndrome (PCOS) and endometriosis. In men, Vitamin D supports sperm health by enhancing sperm motility and reducing oxidative stress in reproductive tissues.

- **Pregnancy Outcomes:** Adequate Vitamin D levels during pregnancy reduce the risk of complications such as preeclampsia, gestational diabetes, and preterm birth. It also supports the healthy development of the fetal brain and immune system.
- **Hormonal Regulation:** Vitamin D influences the production of oestrogen and progesterone, which are crucial for maintaining pregnancy and reproductive cycles in women.

Case History: Samantha, a 32-year-old woman trying to conceive, was found to have low Vitamin D levels. After six months of supplementation, she successfully conceived and had a healthy pregnancy, illustrating the importance of Vitamin D in reproductive health.

9. Respiratory Health: Reducing the Risk of Respiratory Illnesses

Vitamin D's influence on immune function extends to the respiratory system, reducing the risk and severity of respiratory infections and chronic conditions.

- **Asthma Management:** Vitamin D deficiency has been linked to increased asthma severity. Supplementation has been shown to reduce the frequency and severity of asthma attacks by reducing airway inflammation and hypersensitivity.
- **COPD Support:** For individuals with chronic obstructive pulmonary disease (COPD), Vitamin D supplementation has been associated with improved lung function and reduced inflammation.
- **Respiratory Infection Prevention:** Vitamin D helps protect against respiratory infections like the common cold, flu, and pneumonia by enhancing the immune system's ability to fight off pathogens.

Case History: Carlos, a 55-year-old man with COPD, had frequent respiratory infections. After starting Vitamin D supplementation, his infection rate decreased, and his lung function improved, helping him manage his condition more effectively.

10. Skin Health: Enhancing Skin Protection and Healing

Vitamin D plays a critical role in maintaining healthy skin, from promoting wound healing to protecting against skin diseases.

- **Wound Healing:** Vitamin D promotes faster wound healing by regulating the production of key proteins involved in the repair of damaged skin tissue. It also reduces the risk of infection in wounds by boosting local immune responses.
- **Psoriasis Management:** Topical Vitamin D analogues are commonly used to treat psoriasis, a chronic autoimmune condition characterised by scaly skin lesions. Vitamin D reduces the overproduction of skin cells and alleviates inflammation.
- **Acne Control:** Vitamin D's anti-inflammatory properties help reduce acne lesions by regulating sebum production and decreasing the inflammatory response that leads to clogged pores.
- **Sun Protection:** While Vitamin D is synthesised through sun exposure, it also helps protect the skin from UV damage by supporting the body's repair mechanisms.

Case History: Emily, a 28-year-old woman with psoriasis, experienced relief after combining Vitamin D supplementation with topical treatments. Her psoriasis flare-ups were reduced, improving her quality of life.

11. Detoxification: Supporting Liver and Kidney Function

Vitamin D supports the body's detoxification pathways by enhancing the function of organs like the liver and kidneys, which filter toxins from the blood.

- **Liver Health:** Vitamin D plays a role in enhancing liver function by supporting the detoxification of harmful substances. In conditions like non-alcoholic fatty liver disease (NAFLD), higher Vitamin D levels are associated with improved liver enzymes and reduced inflammation.
- **Kidney Health:** In the kidneys, Vitamin D helps regulate calcium and phosphorus balance, preventing kidney stones and reducing the risk of chronic kidney disease.

Case History: John, a 60-year-old man with NAFLD, experienced elevated liver enzymes and fatigue. After starting Vitamin D supplementation, his liver enzymes normalised, and his energy levels improved, demonstrating Vitamin D's role in supporting liver health.

Conclusion:

Vitamin D's influence on human health is profound and far-reaching, with over 101 known ways it supports the body. From maintaining bone density to modulating the immune system, regulating blood pressure, and safeguarding cognitive function, Vitamin D is an essential nutrient for preventing chronic diseases and promoting overall well-being. Correcting Vitamin D deficiency is one of the most effective strategies for enhancing health across multiple systems, ensuring that the body functions optimally at every stage of life

Summary: Vitamin D and scope of support

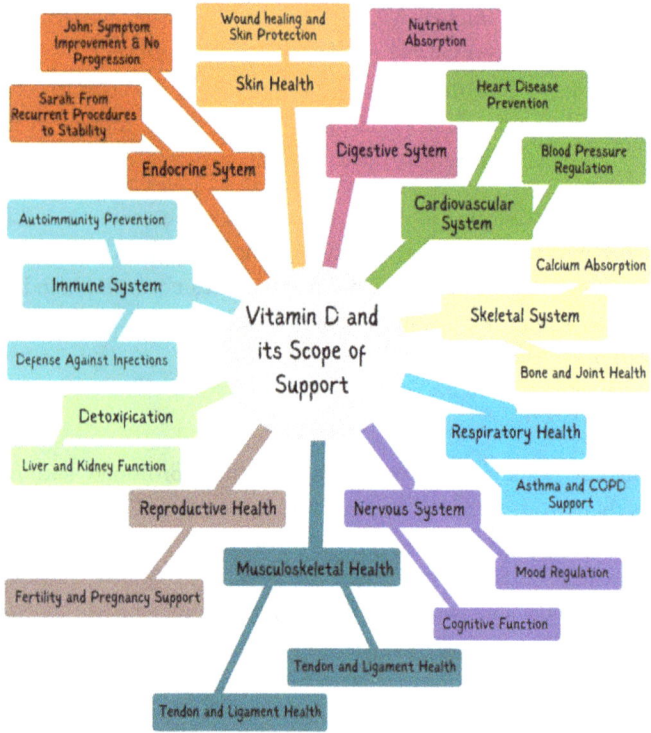

John: Symptom Improvement & No Progression

Sarah: From Recurrent Procedures to Stability

Wound healing and Skin Protection

Skin Health

Nutrient Absorption

Heart Disease Prevention

Blood Pressure Regulation

Digestive Sytem

Endocrine Sytem

Cardiovascular System

Autoimmunity Prevention

Immune System

Defense Against Infections

Calcium Absorption

Skeletal System

Bone and Joint Health

Vitamin D and its Scope of Support

Detoxification

Liver and Kidney Function

Reproductive Health

Nervous System

Respiratory Health

Asthma and COPD Support

Mood Regulation

Fertility and Pregnancy Support

Musculoskeletal Health

Cognitive Function

Tendon and Ligament Health

Tendon and Ligament Health

Chapter 6
Vitamin D Resistance: Why One Size Does Not Fit All

Vitamin D, often referred to as the "sunshine vitamin," is essential for various bodily functions, yet not everyone responds equally to supplementation. The concept of **vitamin D resistance** is increasingly recognised, and it affects millions of individuals globally. This resistance can be attributed to several factors, including genetic mutations, chronic inflammation, environmental influences, and the complex interaction between vitamin D and other hormonal systems. As we learn more, it becomes evident that conventional dosing strategies may be insufficient for certain populations, necessitating more personalised approaches.

Hormonal Interactions and Vitamin D Resistance

Beyond its direct role in calcium homeostasis and immune modulation, vitamin D interacts with other **hormonal systems**, further complicating how it is metabolised and utilised. Understanding these interactions provides deeper insight into why some individuals, particularly those with hormonal imbalances, may experience vitamin D resistance.

Thyroid and Cortisol: Cross-Talk with Vitamin D

Thyroid hormones play a significant role in regulating metabolism, and the thyroid gland itself has **VDRs**, suggesting a link between vitamin D and thyroid function. Patients with **hypothyroidism** or **Hashimoto's thyroiditis**, for example, often present with lower vitamin D levels and may require higher doses of vitamin D to maintain optimal levels. Vitamin D influences thyroid function by modulating the immune system, which is especially critical in autoimmune thyroid disorders.

A study published in the **Endocrine Journal** found that hypothyroid patients supplemented with vitamin D showed improved thyroid function, but individuals with **VDR polymorphisms** such as **TaqI** had a less pronounced response. This suggests that thyroid health and vitamin D metabolism are closely intertwined, and vitamin D resistance in these populations may be partially due to altered hormonal signalling.

In addition to the thyroid, the **cortisol** pathway is closely linked to vitamin D metabolism. Cortisol, a hormone produced by the adrenal glands in response to stress, can negatively influence how the body processes vitamin D. Chronic stress leads to **elevated cortisol levels**, which may downregulate the expression of VDRs, exacerbating vitamin D resistance. Furthermore, high cortisol levels promote inflammation, which, as previously discussed, impairs the conversion of vitamin D into its active form.

A study in **Clinical Endocrinology** suggested that individuals with chronic stress or **Cushing's syndrome** (a condition characterised by excess cortisol) often require both stress management interventions and high-dose vitamin D to overcome resistance. This highlights the need for an integrated approach to treatment, one that considers both hormonal balance and vitamin D status.

Vitamin D and Sex Hormones: Oestrogen and Testosterone

Vitamin D also plays a role in the regulation of **sex hormones**, which further complicates its interaction with different physiological systems. Both **oestrogen** and **testosterone** influence the activity of VDRs, and vitamin D itself can impact the synthesis of these hormones.

In women, oestrogen enhances the expression of VDRs, which explains why **post-menopausal women** often experience vitamin D deficiency and require higher doses for bone health. A study in **Menopause Journal** found that women undergoing oestrogen replacement therapy had improved vitamin D status and bone density, suggesting a synergistic effect between oestrogen and vitamin D. However, women with **polymorphisms in VDR genes** such as **ApaI** showed reduced responsiveness to supplementation, indicating that hormone therapy may not fully overcome genetic resistance.

In men, testosterone is also linked to vitamin D metabolism. Low vitamin D levels have been associated with **hypogonadism** (low testosterone levels), and supplementation can help improve testosterone levels in some cases. A study published in **Andrology** showed that men with low testosterone and vitamin D deficiency required higher doses of vitamin D to restore both hormone levels, particularly if they had VDR mutations that reduced receptor sensitivity.

Epigenetics and Vitamin D: A New Frontier

The interplay between **vitamin D and epigenetics** is an exciting and rapidly evolving area of research. Epigenetics refers to changes in gene expression that occur without altering the underlying DNA sequence, and these changes can be influenced by environmental factors such as diet, stress, and nutrient intake—including vitamin D.

Vitamin D can regulate gene expression by binding to VDRs, which in turn interact with DNA to activate or repress specific genes. However, epigenetic modifications, such as **DNA methylation** or **histone acetylation**, can alter the accessibility of these genes and affect how well vitamin D functions. For example, individuals with certain epigenetic marks on the **VDR gene** may have reduced receptor activity, even in the absence of genetic mutations.

A study published in **Epigenetics Insights** found that individuals with high levels of DNA methylation in the VDR gene had significantly lower responses to vitamin D supplementation, despite adequate intake. The researchers concluded that

epigenetic therapies—such as the use of methyl donors like **folate** or **SAMe**—could potentially "unlock" the VDR and improve responsiveness to vitamin D in resistant individuals.

This line of research opens up exciting possibilities for future treatments, where **personalised supplementation** is not only based on genetic polymorphisms but also on an individual's unique epigenetic profile. Clinicians may one day use **epigenetic testing** alongside genetic testing to fine-tune vitamin D dosing for their patients.

Public Health Perspectives: Rethinking Vitamin D Guidelines

As our understanding of vitamin D resistance grows, it becomes increasingly clear that **public health guidelines** for vitamin D supplementation need to be re-evaluated. Current guidelines often recommend a **one-size-fits-all** approach to vitamin D intake, with standardised dosages aimed at preventing bone diseases such as rickets and osteoporosis. However, this approach does not account for the widespread **individual variability** in vitamin D metabolism.

Rethinking Population-Level Recommendations

A study published in **The Lancet** argued that current vitamin D recommendations are overly conservative and fail to consider the diverse needs of populations with **higher risk factors** for deficiency, such as those with genetic polymorphisms, chronic diseases, or inflammatory conditions. The authors suggested that vitamin D testing should become a routine part of primary care, particularly in populations at higher risk for deficiency, such as the elderly, individuals with autoimmune diseases, and those living in northern latitudes.

Furthermore, the **Endocrine Society** has proposed more aggressive vitamin D supplementation protocols for individuals with chronic diseases, obesity, and other conditions that contribute to vitamin D resistance. These updated guidelines recommend **higher baseline doses** (ranging from 4,000 IU to 10,000 IU daily) for high-risk populations, along with regular testing to monitor blood levels and adjust dosages as necessary.

Practical Approaches for Clinicians

For clinicians, addressing vitamin D resistance requires a **multifaceted approach** that includes both genetic and environmental factors. A personalised strategy might include:

- **Genetic testing** for VDR polymorphisms, particularly in patients with autoimmune diseases or chronic inflammatory conditions.
- **Epigenetic interventions**, such as the use of methyl donors, to modify gene expression and improve VDR activity.
- **Combination therapies**, where vitamin D is paired with supportive nutrients like **magnesium, vitamin K2**, and **omega-3 fatty acids** to enhance absorption and receptor sensitivity.
- **Lifestyle modifications**, such as weight management, stress reduction, and increasing sun exposure, which can improve vitamin D metabolism.

Incorporating these strategies into clinical practice can help overcome resistance and ensure that patients receive the full benefits of vitamin D supplementation.

Conclusion

Vitamin D resistance challenges the conventional understanding of how this critical nutrient is metabolised and utilised in the body. Genetic polymorphisms, epigenetic modifications, hormonal interactions, and environmental factors all contribute to the wide variability in vitamin D responsiveness. To optimise health outcomes, a **personalised approach** to vitamin D supplementation is essential—one that accounts for each individual's unique genetic makeup, health status, and lifestyle factors. As research continues to evolve, clinicians and public health professionals must adapt their strategies to ensure that vitamin D supplementation is tailored to the needs of each individual, particularly in populations at risk for deficiency and resistance.

Summary: Vitamin D Resistance: Why One Size Does Not Fit All

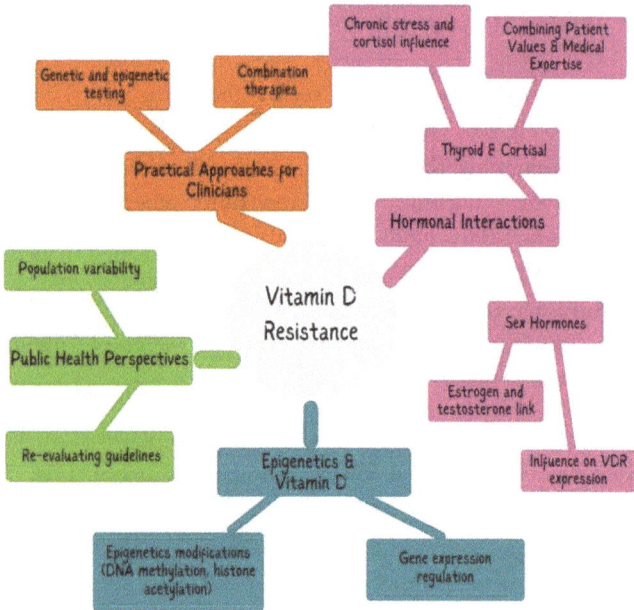

Chapter 7
Mitigating Dementia, MS, and Autoimmunity: A Controversial Approach

Introduction: The Battle Between Innovation and Tradition

Dementia, Multiple Sclerosis (MS), and autoimmune diseases affect millions of individuals globally, leading to severe physical, cognitive, and emotional consequences. While conventional treatments have made progress in managing symptoms, the potential role of high-dose vitamin D in preventing or even reversing these conditions remains a subject of both intrigue and contention. This chapter delves into the scientific evidence supporting the use of high-dose vitamin D protocols, exploring the mechanisms behind vitamin D's potential to slow dementia, halt autoimmune diseases, and reduce chronic inflammation. It also examines why pioneers in the field face resistance from medical authorities, despite growing evidence that natural interventions can complement or surpass pharmacological treatments in certain contexts.

Dementia and Vitamin D: The Sun's Role in Protecting Cognitive Health

Dementia encompasses various forms of cognitive decline, with Alzheimer's disease being the most prevalent. There is a well-established link between vitamin D deficiency and cognitive dysfunction, supported by numerous studies indicating that low levels of vitamin D may accelerate cognitive decline and increase the risk of developing dementia. This association is largely due to vitamin D's neuroprotective properties, which involve several key mechanisms.

Vitamin D exerts its effects on the brain through the presence of vitamin D receptors (VDRs) in neurons and glial cells. These receptors are distributed in regions critical for memory and cognitive function, such as the hippocampus and prefrontal cortex. Upon activation by circulating vitamin D, these receptors modulate various processes that protect the brain from neurodegeneration, including calcium homeostasis, antioxidant activity, and the regulation of neurotrophic factors like nerve growth factor (NGF) and brain-derived neurotrophic factor (BDNF).

One crucial aspect of vitamin D's protective role involves its ability to inhibit the formation and deposition of amyloid-beta plaques, which are characteristic of Alzheimer's disease. A study published in *Springer Link* highlighted how vitamin D enhances the clearance of amyloid-beta peptides by activating macrophages, a type of immune cell that helps clear these toxic aggregates from the brain. Furthermore, vitamin D reduces neuroinflammation by suppressing pro-inflammatory cytokines such as interleukin-6 (IL-6) and tumour necrosis factor-alpha (TNF-alpha), both of which contribute to neuronal damage in Alzheimer's disease.

Additionally, vitamin D's antioxidant properties help mitigate oxidative stress, a key driver of neurodegenerative diseases. By reducing the accumulation of reactive oxygen species (ROS) and promoting the expression of antioxidant enzymes like glutathione peroxidase, vitamin D preserves neuronal integrity and function. This multifaceted neuroprotection suggests that vitamin D sufficiency may play a critical role in delaying the onset of dementia and slowing cognitive decline in affected individuals.

A meta-analysis published in *The Journal of Alzheimer's Disease* demonstrated that individuals with higher baseline levels of vitamin D had a significantly lower risk of developing Alzheimer's and other forms of dementia. These findings suggest that optimising vitamin D levels could be a preventive strategy against cognitive decline, although more large-scale, long-term trials are needed to fully elucidate this relationship.

Multiple Sclerosis: High-Dose Vitamin D and the Immune System

Multiple Sclerosis (MS) is a complex autoimmune disease in which the immune system attacks the myelin sheath surrounding nerve fibres, leading to a range of neurological symptoms. The exact aetiology of MS remains unclear, but vitamin D deficiency has been identified as a major risk factor, particularly in regions with limited sunlight exposure. Vitamin D's role in modulating the immune system makes it a promising candidate for managing MS.

Vitamin D exerts immunomodulatory effects by interacting with VDRs on various immune cells, including T cells, B cells, and dendritic cells. One of the most important actions of vitamin D in the context of autoimmune diseases is its ability to promote the differentiation of regulatory T cells (Tregs). Tregs are critical for maintaining immune tolerance and preventing the immune system from attacking the body's own tissues. In individuals with MS, a deficiency in functional Tregs has been observed, contributing to the uncontrolled immune response that damages myelin.

Vitamin D also inhibits the proliferation of pro-inflammatory Th17 cells, which are implicated in the pathogenesis of MS. Th17 cells produce interleukin-17 (IL-17), a potent pro-inflammatory cytokine that exacerbates neuroinflammation and demyelination in MS. By reducing the activity of Th17 cells and promoting Tregs, vitamin D restores balance in the immune system and reduces the inflammatory attack on myelin.

High-dose vitamin D protocols, such as the Coimbra Protocol, aim to boost serum vitamin D levels to the point where these immunomodulatory effects are maximised. Studies have shown that individuals with MS who receive high doses of vitamin D (often above 10,000 IU/day) exhibit improved neurological function, reduced relapse rates, and lower levels of inflammatory markers in cerebrospinal fluid. One randomised controlled trial published in *Neurology* found that high-dose vitamin D supplementation in MS patients led to a significant reduction in the number of new lesions on MRI scans, suggesting a direct protective effect on the central nervous system.

Although concerns have been raised about the safety of high-dose vitamin D, particularly about hypercalcemia, multiple studies have confirmed that when calcium intake is monitored and kidney function is assessed regularly, high-dose protocols can be safely administered under medical supervision.

Autoimmunity and Inflammation: Targeting the Root Cause of Disease

Vitamin D's influence on the immune system extends beyond MS, with broad applications in the management of autoimmune diseases. Autoimmune diseases occur when the immune system becomes dysregulated, attacking healthy tissues as if they were foreign invaders. This dysregulation is often driven by chronic inflammation, which underlies the pathology of more than 126,000 disease processes, including rheumatoid arthritis, lupus, and type 1 diabetes.

Vitamin D's role in reducing systemic inflammation is well-documented. By inhibiting the production of pro-inflammatory cytokines such as IL-6, TNF-alpha, and interferon-gamma (IFN-gamma), vitamin D interrupts the inflammatory cascade that drives tissue destruction in autoimmune diseases. Furthermore, vitamin D promotes the production of anti-inflammatory cytokines, such as interleukin-10 (IL-10), which help resolve inflammation and restore immune balance.

One key mechanism by which vitamin D reduces inflammation is through its regulation of the NF-kB pathway, a master regulator of the inflammatory response. The NF-kB pathway is activated in response to various stress signals, leading to the expression of genes that promote inflammation. Vitamin D inhibits NF-kB activation, thereby preventing the overproduction of pro-inflammatory molecules that contribute to autoimmune pathogenesis.

In addition to its direct effects on the immune system, vitamin D influences gut health, which is increasingly recognised as a critical factor in autoimmune diseases. The gut microbiome plays a pivotal role in immune regulation, and disruptions to the microbiome are linked to increased intestinal permeability ("leaky gut") and systemic inflammation. Vitamin D helps maintain the integrity of the gut lining by upregulating tight junction proteins, reducing the likelihood of unwanted immune activation by microbial antigens that escape the gut.

A study published in *Frontiers in Immunology* explored the relationship between vitamin D, gut health, and autoimmune disease, concluding that vitamin D supplementation can improve gut barrier function, reduce gut inflammation, and lower the incidence of autoimmune disease flare-ups. These findings support the notion that vitamin D's anti-inflammatory and immunoregulatory properties extend beyond the immune system, influencing broader aspects of human health.

The Suppression of High-Dose Vitamin D Therapy: Vested Interests at Play?

Despite the growing body of evidence supporting high-dose vitamin D therapy, resistance from the medical community and regulatory bodies remains strong. The reasons for this opposition are multifaceted, but one factor that cannot be ignored is the potential threat that inexpensive, natural interventions like vitamin D pose to the pharmaceutical industry. Chronic diseases, especially autoimmune diseases, represent a major revenue stream for pharmaceutical companies, with patients often requiring lifelong medication to manage their symptoms. In contrast, vitamin D is a low-cost, widely available nutrient with the potential to reduce reliance on costly medications.

Several high-profile figures in the field of vitamin D research, including Dr Cicero Coimbra, Dr Michael Holick, and Dr Terry Wahls, have faced professional reprimand for promoting high-dose vitamin D protocols. Their experiences highlight the challenges of advocating for natural therapies that challenge the dominance of pharmaceutical solutions. Despite these challenges, the scientific evidence continues to mount, suggesting that vitamin D may be an invaluable tool in the fight against dementia, MS, and autoimmune diseases.

Conclusion: The Path Forward for High-Dose Vitamin D Therapy

As the understanding of vitamin D's biological functions continues to expand, its role in managing and potentially curing conditions like dementia, MS, and autoimmune diseases is becoming increasingly clear. While high-dose vitamin D therapy remains controversial, the scientific evidence supporting its efficacy is compelling, and the benefits it offers in reducing inflammation, modulating the immune system, and protecting the brain are undeniable.

The reluctance of medical authorities to fully embrace high-dose vitamin D protocols speaks to the broader issue of how natural, cost-effective interventions are often sidelined in favour of pharmaceutical treatments. However, with continued research and growing patient advocacy, the tide may shift in favour of holistic, vitamin D-based approaches to health.

Summary: Mitigating Dementia, MS, and Autoimmunity: A Controversial Approach

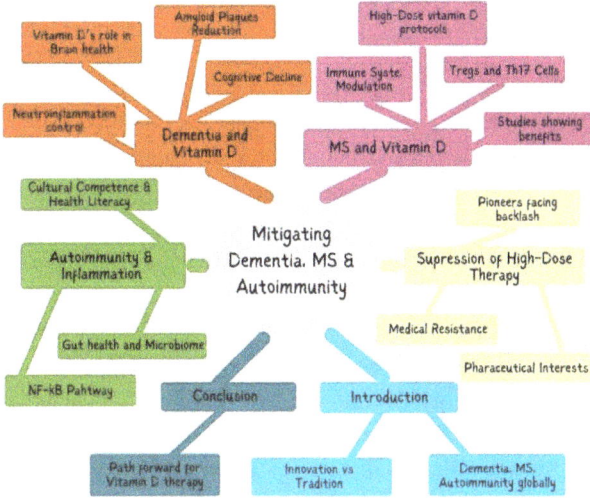

Chapter 8
Challenging Conventional Guidelines

Vitamin D is widely recognised as one of the most critical nutrients for human health, yet its recommended daily intake (RDA) remains surprisingly low, leading many experts to consider it grossly inadequate. The current guidelines, which suggest a daily intake of 600–800 IU, are primarily aimed at preventing rickets and other skeletal disorders. However, these recommendations overlook the broader roles of vitamin D in immune function, cardiovascular health, neurological processes, and chronic disease prevention. This chapter delves into the reasons why the current RDA limits are outdated and why health organisations have been reluctant to update them despite the accumulating body of evidence. It also explores the consequences of these outdated guidelines on public health.

Current RDA Limitations: Why the 600-800 IU/day Recommendation is Outdated

The recommended daily allowance for vitamin D, which stands at 600–800 IU, was established decades ago with a narrow focus on skeletal health. It was based on the minimum amount needed to prevent rickets and ensure adequate bone mineralisation. While these goals are important, they represent only a small fraction of vitamin D's physiological roles. Over the past few decades, research has revealed vitamin D's involvement in numerous critical functions, far beyond bone health, highlighting the inadequacies of the current guidelines.

The Expanding Role of Vitamin D in Human Health

Vitamin D functions as more than just a vitamin; it acts like a hormone, regulating a wide array of biological processes. One of the most striking revelations in recent years is the discovery that vitamin D receptors (VDRs) are present in nearly every tissue and cell in the human body. This finding underscores its vast influence on systems such as the immune, cardiovascular, and nervous systems. Vitamin D's role in modulating the immune response, for example, is critical for preventing autoimmune diseases like multiple sclerosis (MS), lupus, and rheumatoid arthritis.

A landmark study published in *The Journal of Clinical Endocrinology & Metabolism* demonstrated that vitamin D levels significantly above the current RDA are required to support the immune system and protect against chronic diseases. In fact, the study found that individuals with serum 25(OH)D levels above 50 ng/mL had significantly lower risks of developing autoimmune and cardiovascular conditions compared to those with lower levels.

Moreover, emerging evidence suggests that optimal vitamin D levels can help prevent a range of chronic illnesses, from heart disease to type 2 diabetes. Research has also linked higher vitamin D levels to improved mood and cognitive function, emphasising its importance in brain health. However, achieving these protective levels often requires a daily intake well above the 600–800 IU currently recommended, sometimes in the range of 4,000 IU or more.

The Global Epidemic of Vitamin D Deficiency

One of the key arguments against the current RDA is that it leaves a significant portion of the global population at risk of vitamin D deficiency. According to a report by the *International Journal of Environmental Research and Public Health*, approximately 1 billion people worldwide are deficient in vitamin D, while another 50% have insufficient levels. This widespread deficiency cannot be explained by individual factors alone, such as skin colour or geographic location; it is also a consequence of outdated recommendations that do not reflect modern lifestyles or the growing understanding of vitamin D's roles.

At the current RDA, many people, particularly those living in northern latitudes or those with darker skin, do not produce enough vitamin D from sunlight alone and require supplementation. The problem is exacerbated by modern indoor lifestyles, which limit sun exposure, making it nearly impossible to achieve adequate vitamin D levels without significant supplementation. For instance, a study in *Nutrients* found that even individuals who adhered to the 600–800 IU RDA were often still deficient, particularly during the winter months when sunlight was scarce.

RDA Based on Skeletal Health Alone

The focus on bone health alone when setting the current RDA for vitamin D is a significant limitation. While skeletal health is important, it represents only a small part of what vitamin D does in the body. The fixation on preventing rickets or osteoporosis has overshadowed the broader benefits that higher levels of vitamin D can provide. Research in *The Journal of the American Medical Association* (JAMA) suggests that achieving higher vitamin D levels—closer to 50–60 ng/mL—offers substantial protection against respiratory infections, autoimmune diseases, and even certain cancers.

This disconnect between the skeletal focus of the current RDA and the expanding understanding of vitamin D's role in overall health is one of the main reasons why the recommendations are increasingly viewed as inadequate. An intake of 600–800 IU may prevent rickets, but it does not address the needs of the immune system, heart, or brain. To optimise health in the modern world, many experts now recommend daily intakes of 2,000–4,000 IU or more, especially in individuals who have limited sun exposure or other risk factors for deficiency.

The Growing Consensus for Higher Vitamin D Intake

The scientific consensus on vitamin D has shifted dramatically over the past two decades, with an increasing number of researchers and clinicians advocating for higher daily intakes. For example, the Endocrine Society suggests that adults require at least 1,500–2,000 IU of vitamin D per day to maintain optimal health. This recommendation is based on extensive studies showing that higher intakes are needed to achieve serum 25(OH)D levels of 40–60 ng/mL, which are associated with a reduced risk of chronic diseases.

A systematic review published in *The American Journal of Clinical Nutrition* further supports the need for higher intake, concluding that higher vitamin D levels are associated with improved immune function and a lower risk of chronic diseases. Despite these findings, health organisations such as the National Institutes of Health (NIH) and the Institute of Medicine (IOM) have been slow to update their guidelines.

Resistance to Change: Health Organisations' Reluctance to Update Vitamin D Guidelines

Despite the compelling evidence for higher vitamin D intake, health organisations have been remarkably slow to revise their recommendations. Several factors contribute to this resistance to change, including concerns about safety, institutional inertia, and the influence of vested interests. This section explores these reasons in more detail and examines why outdated guidelines continue to persist.

Fear of Toxicity: A Misguided Concern

One of the most common reasons cited for maintaining low RDA levels is the concern over vitamin D toxicity. Since vitamin D is fat-soluble, it is stored in the body, and excessively high levels can lead to hypercalcemia, a condition in which calcium levels in the blood become dangerously high. This condition can cause kidney stones, cardiovascular issues, and even death in extreme cases. However, vitamin D toxicity is exceedingly rare and typically only occurs at doses well above 10,000 IU/day taken over prolonged periods.

A study published in *The New England Journal of Medicine* found that even at doses of up to 10,000 IU/day, most individuals experienced no adverse effects, and toxicity was almost exclusively associated with intakes exceeding 50,000 IU/day for several months. Nevertheless, concerns over toxicity persist, largely due to outdated safety data that health organisations continue to rely on.

This overly cautious approach has hindered progress in updating vitamin D guidelines, despite evidence showing that higher doses are not only safe but also necessary for optimal health. By clinging to concerns about toxicity, health organisations are preventing millions of people from reaping the full benefits of adequate vitamin D intake.

Skeletal-Centric Viewpoint: An Outdated Paradigm

Another reason for the resistance to updating vitamin D guidelines is that many health organisations continue to focus narrowly on its role in bone health. When vitamin D was first discovered, its primary function was believed to be the regulation of calcium and phosphate levels for bone mineralisation. This view dominated public health policy for decades, leading to guidelines that prioritised skeletal health while ignoring vitamin D's broader functions.

This narrow perspective has persisted in many health organisations, even as new research has revealed the vitamin's extensive influence on other systems. For example, vitamin D has been shown to regulate the expression of genes involved in immune function, inflammation, and cellular differentiation. A meta-analysis in *The BMJ* concluded that vitamin D supplementation significantly reduces the risk of acute respiratory infections and other inflammatory conditions, yet these findings have not prompted a meaningful change in the guidelines.

Institutional Inertia and Bureaucratic Hurdles

Institutional inertia also plays a significant role in the reluctance to update vitamin D guidelines. Large health organisations like the NIH, IOM, and World Health Organisation (WHO) are notoriously slow-moving, especially when it comes to implementing new recommendations that affect public health policy. These institutions must consider a range of factors, including potential risks, costs, and political pressures, all of which can delay the adoption of new guidelines.

In addition, public health agencies are often influenced by pharmaceutical companies, which have little incentive to promote higher vitamin D intake. Since vitamin D is inexpensive and widely available as a supplement, increasing public awareness of its benefits could reduce reliance on more expensive pharmaceuticals, which could hurt the bottom lines of major pharmaceutical companies. According to a report in *Public Health Nutrition*, financial ties between pharmaceutical companies and health organisations may play a role in the reluctance to endorse higher vitamin D intakes.

The Path Forward: Revising Guidelines for a Healthier Future

While resistance from health organisations persists, there is a clear and urgent need to revise vitamin D guidelines to reflect current scientific understanding. Updating the RDA to higher levels could have profound effects on public health, reducing the burden of chronic diseases and improving overall well-being. Moreover, increasing public awareness of vitamin D's broader health benefits is essential for empowering individuals to take control of their health.

Advocacy and Education

Several organisations and researchers are advocating for higher vitamin D intake and working to change outdated guidelines. The

Vitamin D Council, for example, recommends daily intakes of at least 5,000 IU, based on the latest scientific research. Similarly, the Endocrine Society has called for higher intake recommendations, emphasising that the current RDA is insufficient for most people.

Education is another key factor in shifting public health policy. By increasing awareness of vitamin D's broader health benefits, particularly its role in immune modulation and chronic disease prevention, individuals can make informed decisions about their supplementation needs. Health organisations should also work to make vitamin D supplements more accessible and affordable, particularly for at-risk populations.

Addressing Safety Concerns

To address safety concerns, health organisations must update their understanding of vitamin D toxicity. The evidence overwhelmingly supports the safety of daily intakes well above the current RDA, and fears of toxicity are largely unfounded at moderate to high doses. By providing clear guidance on safe upper limits—such as 10,000 IU/day—public health agencies can encourage individuals to achieve optimal vitamin D levels without fear of adverse effects.

Summary: Challenging Conventional Guidelines

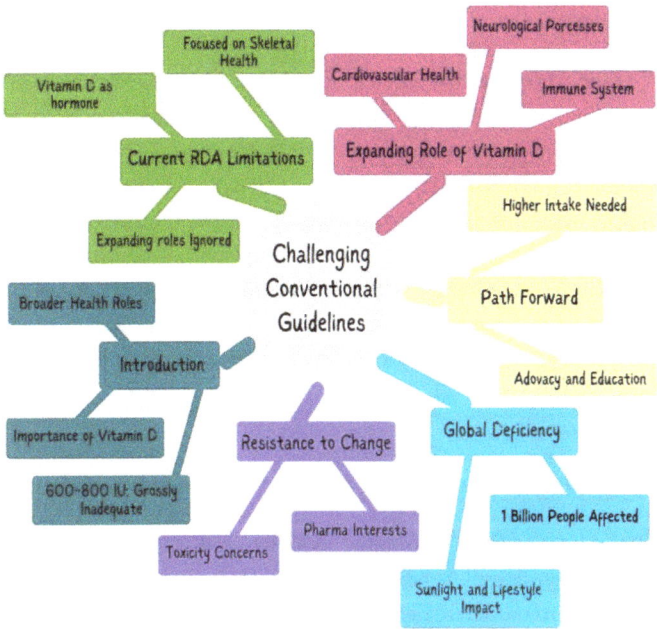

Chapter 9
Methods of Administering Vitamin D

Introduction

Vitamin D is essential for a wide array of physiological processes, including bone health, immune regulation, and even mood stabilisation. As deficiencies in vitamin D have become more common globally, ensuring adequate levels through supplementation has become a priority. The methods of vitamin D administration—oral, sublingual, and injectable—each come with their own sets of benefits and limitations. In this chapter, we will explore these methods, along with the importance of regular monitoring, and highlight research that supports the use of injectable vitamin D in cases of severe deficiency or poor absorption.

Oral Administration: The Most Common Method

Oral vitamin D is the most popular and accessible method. Available in capsules, tablets, and liquids, it is a go-to for people with mild to moderate deficiencies.

Advantages of Oral Vitamin D:

- **Convenience:** Oral supplements are widely available, with various doses to suit individual needs.

- **Cost-effectiveness:** Oral supplementation is often cheaper than other methods.

- **Consistency:** For individuals without significant health issues affecting absorption, oral vitamin D can be effective.

Disadvantages of Oral Vitamin D:

- **Variable Absorption:** Studies like those by *Cavalier et al. (2017)* show that oral vitamin D absorption can be inconsistent due to factors like gut health, age, or fat intake. People with conditions such as Crohn's disease or celiac disease may experience inadequate absorption.

Sublingual Administration: Bypassing the Gut

Sublingual vitamin D, which involves placing drops or tablets under the tongue, allows for direct absorption into the bloodstream, bypassing the digestive tract.

Advantages of Sublingual Vitamin D:

- **Improved Absorption:** By bypassing the digestive system, sublingual administration can improve vitamin D absorption, particularly for individuals with gastrointestinal issues.
- **Faster Action:** Sublingual methods deliver vitamin D into the bloodstream more rapidly than oral supplements, which is beneficial when a quicker boost in levels is needed.

Disadvantages:

- **Limited Availability:** Sublingual forms are less widely available than oral supplements.
- **Dosing Challenges:** Adjusting doses may be harder with sublingual forms, especially in individuals requiring high doses.

Injectable Vitamin D: The Superior Solution

Injectable vitamin D is a potent solution for individuals with severe deficiencies or chronic absorption issues. It offers rapid correction of vitamin D levels and long-lasting effects, making it particularly effective for people who cannot absorb vitamin D adequately through oral or sublingual methods.

Advantages of Injectable Vitamin D:

- **Rapid Effect:** Research by *Glendenning et al. (2012)* demonstrates that injectable vitamin D rapidly increases serum 25(OH)D levels more efficiently than oral doses, particularly in individuals with severe deficiency.
- **Sustained Levels:** Injectable vitamin D maintains elevated blood levels for longer periods, reducing the frequency of doses required. This was reinforced by *Glendenning et al.* who found that a single high-dose injection sustained vitamin D levels significantly better than weekly oral supplementation.
- **Solves Malabsorption Issues:** For people with conditions that impair nutrient absorption, such as Crohn's disease, bariatric surgery, or celiac disease, injectable vitamin D offers a reliable solution.

Disadvantages:

- **Invasiveness:** Injections are more invasive and need to be administered by a healthcare professional, which could be a barrier for some patients.
- **Cost and Access:** Injectable vitamin D may be more expensive and less accessible than oral or sublingual forms.

Research Evidence Supporting Injectable Vitamin D

Several key studies have demonstrated the superiority of injectable vitamin D for addressing deficiencies, especially in individuals with severe or chronic conditions.

1. **Faster Correction of Deficiencies:** Injectable vitamin D has been shown to correct deficiencies more quickly than oral or sublingual supplements. *Cavalier et al. (2017)* highlighted that, while oral supplementation is generally effective for mild deficiencies, injectable forms are more effective in rapidly increasing serum 25(OH)D levels in individuals with severe deficiencies or malabsorption syndromes. This rapid correction is crucial in conditions like osteomalacia or

autoimmune disorders, where timely intervention can prevent further health deterioration.

2. **Sustained Blood Levels:** A randomised controlled trial by *Glendenning et al. (2012)* demonstrated that a single high-dose injection of vitamin D3 maintained higher and more stable serum 25(OH)D levels compared to weekly or monthly oral doses in older women with vitamin D insufficiency. This long-lasting effect reduces the need for frequent supplementation, making injections more convenient for long-term management of vitamin D deficiency.

3. **Better Symptom Control:** A review by *Kearns et al. (2015)* on the impact of vitamin D on skeletal muscle function found that patients receiving injectable vitamin D reported significant improvements in muscle strength and performance compared to oral supplements. Similarly, individuals suffering from chronic fatigue syndrome saw marked improvement in symptoms after receiving vitamin D injections. *Pierrot-Deseilligny et al. (2017)* also demonstrated that patients with multiple sclerosis (MS) treated with high-dose injectable vitamin D experienced fewer relapses and better disease management than those on oral supplementation, highlighting the broader immune-regulatory benefits of injections.

Monitoring and Optimal Levels

Whether using oral, sublingual, or injectable forms, maintaining optimal vitamin D levels is key. Regular monitoring ensures levels stay within the ideal range of **175-200 nmol/L** to avoid both deficiency and toxicity.

For Oral and Sublingual Administration: Testing is recommended every 3-6 months until optimal levels are reached. Once stabilised, monitoring can be reduced to every 6 months. If levels rise too high, adjustments should be made to avoid toxicity.

For Injections: Since injectable vitamin D raises blood levels more rapidly, testing is recommended every 1-3 months initially, especially in cases of severe deficiency. Once levels stabilise between **175-200 nmol/L**, testing every 6 months is sufficient.

Conclusion: Tailoring Vitamin D Treatment

Selecting the right method of administering vitamin D depends on the severity of the deficiency, individual health conditions, and personal preferences. While oral supplementation is widely accessible and effective for many, sublingual and injectable methods offer significant advantages for individuals with absorption issues or severe deficiencies.

Research, including studies by *Cavalier et al. (2017)*, *Glendenning et al. (2012)*, *Kearns et al. (2015)*, and *Pierrot-Deseilligny et al. (2017)*, consistently supports the rapid and sustained benefits of injectable vitamin D. Injectable forms not only raise blood levels faster but also maintain them over longer periods, making them ideal for individuals needing immediate correction and long-term maintenance. As more is learned about the broad health implications of vitamin D, ensuring optimal levels through the most appropriate administration method remains crucial to achieving long-term health benefits.

Summary: Methods of Administering Vitamin D

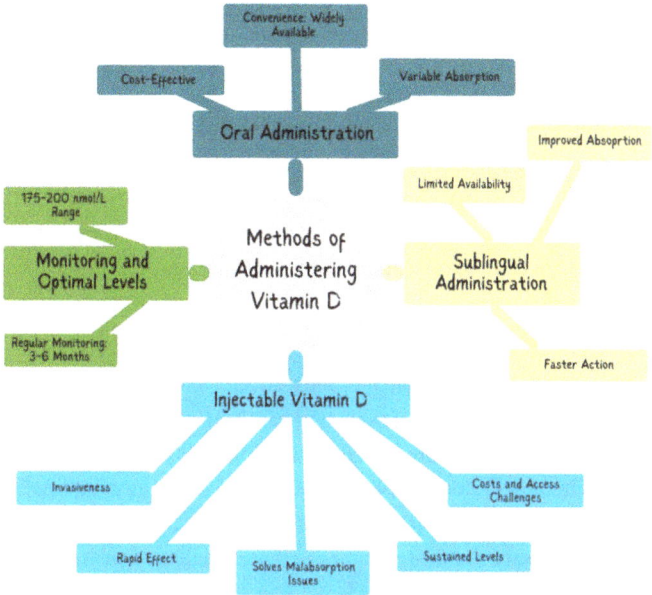

Chapter 10
Debunking the Myths
Around Vitamin D

Vitamin D is one of the most researched vitamins, yet its benefits remain misunderstood. Misinformation abounds regarding its safety, efficacy, and the best ways to obtain adequate levels. This chapter aims to dismantle some of the most persistent myths surrounding vitamin D, using scientific evidence to clarify the truths behind these misconceptions.

Myth 1: High-Dose Toxicity — Evidence Showing Safety

One of the most prevalent myths about vitamin D is that high doses are inherently dangerous and can lead to toxicity. This belief has led many healthcare providers and patients to avoid increasing their vitamin D levels, even when deficient. However, research shows that vitamin D toxicity is extremely rare, and high doses are often necessary for those who are severely deficient or have higher metabolic demands.

Vitamin D toxicity, also known as hypervitaminosis D, occurs when there are excessively high levels of vitamin D in the body, leading to elevated calcium levels (hypercalcemia), which can cause nausea, vomiting, weakness, and in severe cases, kidney problems. However, studies show that this toxicity is only seen in individuals consuming **over 10,000 IU/day** for extended periods, usually over several months. The Institute of Medicine (IOM) has set the upper tolerable intake level for adults at **4,000 IU/day**, but many researchers argue this figure is conservative, especially given the increasing prevalence of deficiency.

A study published in the **Journal of Clinical Endocrinology & Metabolism** showed that patients taking **up to 10,000 IU/day** of vitamin D over five months had no signs of toxicity or adverse health effects. Additionally, a randomised controlled trial reported in **MDPI** demonstrated that daily doses of **5,000-8,000 IU** were safe and effective in maintaining optimal serum vitamin D levels without adverse effects.

Critics of high-dose vitamin D supplementation often point to hypercalcemia as a risk. However, it is important to note that vitamin D alone does not automatically cause calcium imbalances. In fact, hypercalcemia is often a result of underlying conditions such as **hyperparathyroidism** or **renal dysfunction**, rather than vitamin D supplementation itself. Therefore, toxicity is exceedingly rare and typically occurs only when extremely high doses are paired with calcium-rich diets or pre-existing health conditions that affect calcium regulation.

For individuals with **autoimmune diseases**, chronic inflammation, or **vitamin D resistance**, higher doses may be essential to achieve therapeutic outcomes. Research published in **Springer Link** further supports the safety of **high-dose vitamin D** in patients with chronic illnesses, demonstrating that dosing regimens of **up to 50,000 IU weekly** can be safely administered under medical supervision to correct deficiencies.

Myth 2: Dietary Sufficiency — Why Sunlight and Supplements Are Crucial

Another persistent myth is that people can get enough vitamin D through diet alone. While certain foods such as fatty fish (salmon, mackerel), fortified dairy products, and egg yolks do contain vitamin D, the amounts are often too small to meet daily needs, especially in individuals with higher demands or those living in regions with low sun exposure.

For example, a typical serving of salmon contains about **400 IU** of vitamin D, while an egg yolk provides just **40 IU**. Given that the recommended daily allowance (RDA) for vitamin D is **600 IU for adults**, and this figure is often considered **insufficient for optimal health**, it is clear that food sources alone cannot provide adequate levels for most individuals. Furthermore, for individuals with health conditions that impact vitamin D metabolism—such as obesity, chronic kidney disease, or gastrointestinal disorders—dietary intake is often inadequate to correct deficiencies.

Sunlight is the most efficient and natural source of vitamin D. When UVB rays from the sun hit the skin, they trigger the production of vitamin D3, the most bioavailable form of the vitamin. However, **modern lifestyles**, including long hours indoors, the use of sunscreen, and living in regions with **limited sunlight**, have significantly reduced our ability to produce adequate vitamin D naturally. In addition, **people with darker skin** require longer sun exposure to produce the same amount of vitamin D as those with lighter skin due to the higher levels of melanin, which absorbs UVB rays.

A study published in **MDPI** revealed that **70% of the global population** is either vitamin D deficient or insufficient due to the combined effects of low dietary intake and limited sun exposure. The study emphasised the importance of **supplementation** to close this gap and reduce the burden of deficiency-related diseases such as osteoporosis, cardiovascular diseases, and autoimmune conditions.

Recent clinical guidelines also stress the importance of vitamin D supplements, particularly in regions where **UVB exposure is minimal for parts of the year**, such as in Northern Europe and Canada. Researchers from **Springer Link** highlighted the limitations of relying on food sources for vitamin D and recommended routine supplementation as the most effective strategy for maintaining optimal levels throughout the year.

Myth 3: Only the Elderly Need Vitamin D Supplements

A common misconception is that only the elderly need to worry about vitamin D supplementation because they are at higher risk for osteoporosis. While it is true that **bone health** is a key concern in ageing populations, vitamin D plays a crucial role in many other physiological processes that affect individuals of all ages. From

immune system modulation to **cardiovascular health** and **mental well-being**, vitamin D is essential for maintaining overall health across the lifespan.

Children, for example, are at risk of **rickets**, a condition caused by vitamin D deficiency, which leads to soft, weak bones. While rickets have become less common in many parts of the world due to fortification programs, they remain a concern in certain regions, particularly in communities with **low sun exposure** and **limited access to fortified foods**. Moreover, research shows that children require **higher doses** of vitamin D than previously thought, especially during periods of rapid growth and immune system development. According to a study published in **MDPI**, supplementing children with **1,000 IU/day** of vitamin D significantly reduced the risk of respiratory infections and improved overall immune function.

Additionally, individuals with **autoimmune diseases**, such as multiple sclerosis (MS) or type 1 diabetes, may have an increased need for vitamin D to regulate immune function and reduce inflammation. Vitamin D's role in **immune modulation** is well-documented, and its deficiency has been linked to **increased susceptibility** to infections and chronic inflammatory conditions across all age groups.

Pregnant women also require adequate vitamin D to support **fetal development** and **reduce the risk of complications** such as preeclampsia and gestational diabetes. A review published in **Springer Link** showed that pregnant women who were supplemented with **4,000 IU/day** of vitamin D had significantly better pregnancy outcomes than those who followed the standard RDA of 600 IU.

Myth 4: Vitamin D is Only Important for Bone Health

Although vitamin D is best known for its role in **calcium absorption** and **bone health**, its impact goes far beyond the skeletal system. In recent years, research has uncovered the

multifaceted functions of vitamin D, including its effects on the **immune system**, **cardiovascular health**, and **mental health**.

Vitamin D is a powerful immune modulator, meaning it helps regulate the immune response to prevent both **infections** and **autoimmune diseases**. For example, studies have shown that vitamin D deficiency is associated with an increased risk of **respiratory infections**, including the common cold and influenza. A meta-analysis published in the **British Medical Journal** found that regular vitamin D supplementation reduced the risk of respiratory tract infections by **12%**, especially in individuals with low baseline levels.

Moreover, vitamin D has been linked to **cardiovascular health**, with deficiencies contributing to conditions such as hypertension, atherosclerosis, and heart disease. A study published in **Springer Link** demonstrated that individuals with **low vitamin D levels** had a higher risk of developing cardiovascular diseases compared to those with adequate levels. The researchers concluded that maintaining optimal vitamin D levels through supplementation could reduce the risk of heart disease and improve overall cardiovascular function.

In the realm of **mental health**, vitamin D has been shown to play a role in regulating **mood** and reducing the risk of depression. A study published in **MDPI** revealed that individuals with vitamin D deficiency were more likely to experience **depressive symptoms**, while supplementation improved mood and reduced anxiety.

Conclusion

The myths surrounding vitamin D have contributed to widespread misinformation and have prevented many people from achieving optimal health. As the evidence shows, vitamin D toxicity is rare, and high-dose supplementation is often safe and necessary for correcting deficiencies. Additionally, relying solely on dietary sources is insufficient for most people, and supplementation is crucial for maintaining adequate levels. Beyond bone health, vitamin D plays a vital role in immune regulation, cardiovascular health, and mental well-being, making it an essential nutrient for individuals of all ages. By debunking these myths, we can better understand the importance of vitamin D and take proactive steps to protect our health.

Summary: Debunking the Myths Around Vitamin D

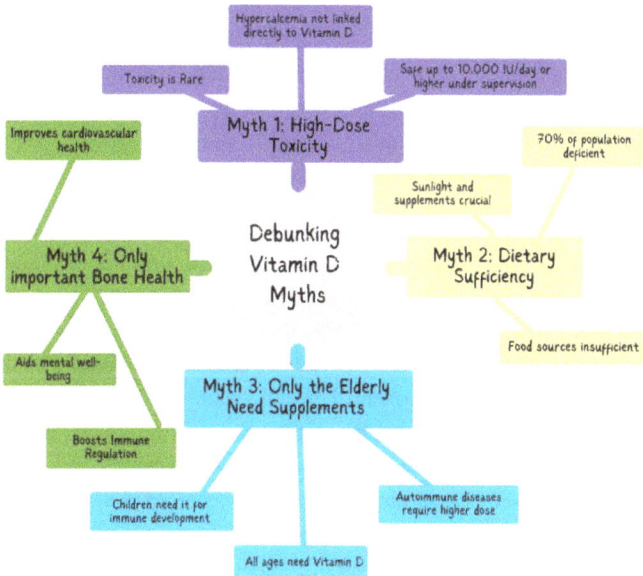

Chapter 11
The Future of Vitamin D in Medicine

Vitamin D has long been recognised for its essential role in bone health and calcium regulation. However, emerging research in recent years has expanded our understanding of this vital nutrient, revealing its potential in several critical areas of medicine, including mental health, cancer prevention, and cardiovascular care. As we dive into these new domains, the public health implications of optimising vitamin D levels become increasingly significant. This chapter explores the future of vitamin D in medicine, highlighting groundbreaking studies and potential shifts in public health recommendations that could shape how we approach this vital hormone in the years to come.

Emerging Research: Vitamin D's Role in Mental Health

One of the most exciting areas of emerging research is the potential role of vitamin D in mental health. Traditionally associated with musculoskeletal health, vitamin D is now being explored for its effects on brain function and mood regulation. Studies have shown a correlation between low levels of vitamin D and an increased risk of mood disorders, including depression and anxiety. This connection is thought to stem from vitamin D's involvement in the synthesis of neurotransmitters, including serotonin, which plays a crucial role in regulating mood.

A growing body of evidence supports the hypothesis that vitamin D deficiency may be a contributing factor to the onset of mental health disorders. A meta-analysis published in *MDPI* in 2022 examined the link between vitamin D levels and depression, concluding that individuals with low levels of vitamin D are significantly more likely to experience depressive symptoms. Moreover, supplementation with vitamin D has been shown to improve mood in individuals who are deficient, suggesting that maintaining optimal levels of vitamin D may serve as a preventative measure against certain mood disorders.

Beyond depression, vitamin D is being investigated for its potential in neurodevelopmental disorders such as autism and ADHD. Some studies indicate that adequate vitamin D levels during pregnancy may lower the risk of autism spectrum disorders in offspring. Furthermore, research published in *Frontiers in Neuroscience* has explored how vitamin D's role in reducing neuroinflammation may contribute to improved outcomes in conditions like multiple sclerosis, a disease with both neurological and immunological dimensions.

While much remains to be understood about the precise mechanisms, the growing interest in vitamin D as a modulator of brain health suggests it may become a key player in future mental health interventions. As ongoing clinical trials continue to explore this area, vitamin D's role in mood regulation and neurological health may soon gain mainstream acceptance in clinical practice.

Cancer Prevention: A New Frontier for Vitamin D

The relationship between vitamin D and cancer prevention has been an area of significant research over the past few decades. Vitamin D's anti-cancer potential is largely attributed to its ability to regulate cell growth, apoptosis (programmed cell death), and differentiation. These properties are particularly important in preventing the uncontrolled growth characteristic of cancer cells.

Research published in *Frontiers in Oncology* highlights the emerging evidence linking adequate vitamin D levels with a reduced risk of various cancers, including breast, colorectal, and prostate cancer. Vitamin D's role in cancer prevention appears to be multi-faceted, involving the modulation of gene expression and the immune response. The active form of vitamin D, calcitriol, is known to influence the expression of genes involved in cell cycle regulation and tumour suppression. Furthermore, vitamin D enhances the immune system's ability to identify and destroy cancer cells by increasing the activity of natural killer cells and macrophages.

A 2021 study published in *MDPI* examined the relationship between vitamin D status and cancer outcomes, finding that individuals with higher serum levels of vitamin D had significantly lower mortality rates in various cancer types. These findings are particularly promising, as they suggest that vitamin D may not only help prevent cancer but also improve survival rates among those diagnosed with the disease.

However, despite the promising data, the use of vitamin D as a cancer-preventive agent is still a topic of debate within the medical community. While observational studies have consistently shown a protective effect, randomised controlled trials (RCTs) have yielded more mixed results. Some researchers argue that the variation in outcomes may be due to differences in baseline vitamin D levels among study participants or insufficient dosages in supplementation trials. As more well-designed RCTs are conducted, the potential for vitamin D to play a role in cancer prevention and treatment will become clearer.

Cardiovascular Care: Vitamin D's Expanding Influence

The role of vitamin D in cardiovascular health is another rapidly evolving area of research. While traditionally associated with bone and immune health, vitamin D has also been found to influence heart function and vascular health. Studies have demonstrated that vitamin D deficiency is linked to an increased risk of hypertension, atherosclerosis, and heart failure. These findings are significant, given the global burden of cardiovascular disease as a leading cause of mortality.

Vitamin D's effect on cardiovascular health is thought to be mediated through several mechanisms. First, vitamin D plays a role in regulating blood pressure by modulating the renin-angiotensin-aldosterone system (RAAS), a hormone system that controls blood pressure and fluid balance. By inhibiting renin production, vitamin D helps to lower blood pressure and reduce the risk of hypertension. Additionally, vitamin D has anti-inflammatory properties, which may protect the cardiovascular system from the chronic inflammation that contributes to the development of atherosclerosis.

Research published in *Frontiers in Cardiovascular Medicine* in 2020 found that individuals with higher vitamin D levels had a lower risk of developing heart disease and related complications. Furthermore, supplementation with vitamin D in deficient individuals has been shown to improve endothelial function, which is critical for maintaining the elasticity of blood vessels and preventing the formation of plaques that can lead to heart attacks or strokes.

Despite these promising findings, the role of vitamin D in cardiovascular care remains somewhat controversial. Some studies have failed to show a clear benefit of supplementation in reducing cardiovascular events, leading to calls for more targeted research. Factors such as dosage, baseline vitamin D status, and individual differences in metabolism may all influence the outcomes of these studies. As research continues, vitamin D may eventually become a routine part of cardiovascular disease prevention and treatment protocols.

Shaping Public Health: New Recommendations for Vitamin D

As our understanding of vitamin D's broader health impacts grows, there is increasing pressure to update public health recommendations to reflect the latest research. Current guidelines for vitamin D intake, set by organisations such as the Institute of Medicine (IOM) and the Endocrine Society, primarily focus on bone health and recommend daily intakes of 600-800 IU for most adults. However, these recommendations are based on preventing bone-related conditions such as rickets and osteoporosis and do not account for vitamin D's potential in other areas of health.

A growing number of experts argue that current guidelines are outdated and insufficient to address the wide range of health issues linked to vitamin D deficiency. Research suggests that optimal vitamin D levels for preventing chronic diseases, such as cancer and cardiovascular disease, may be much higher than those needed for bone health alone. For instance, many studies indicate that maintaining serum levels of 25-hydroxyvitamin D above 30 ng/mL is necessary for reducing the risk of chronic diseases, whereas current guidelines recommend a minimum level of 20 ng/mL.

Public health initiatives aimed at increasing awareness of vitamin D deficiency are already underway in several countries. In the United Kingdom, for example, the National Health Service (NHS) has recommended that individuals take vitamin D supplements, particularly during the winter months when sunlight exposure is limited. Similarly, in Scandinavian countries, food fortification programs have been implemented to increase the population's vitamin D intake.

As more research emerges, we are likely to see further shifts in public health recommendations. Organisations such as *MDPI* and *Frontiers* continue to publish studies that highlight the need for higher vitamin D intake to support overall health, particularly in populations at risk of deficiency. With growing recognition of vitamin D's role in preventing chronic diseases, future guidelines may emphasise higher daily intake levels and routine monitoring of vitamin D status as part of standard medical care.

Conclusion: A Bright Future for Vitamin D

The future of vitamin D in medicine is promising. As new research sheds light on its role in mental health, cancer prevention, and cardiovascular care, the potential for vitamin D to become a cornerstone of preventative medicine grows. However, much work remains to be done. The medical community must continue to investigate the optimal levels of vitamin D for different health outcomes and ensure that public health recommendations are updated to reflect the latest science. With its far-reaching effects on health, vitamin D is poised to play a pivotal role in shaping the future of medicine and public health policy.

Summary: The Future of Vitamin D in Medicine

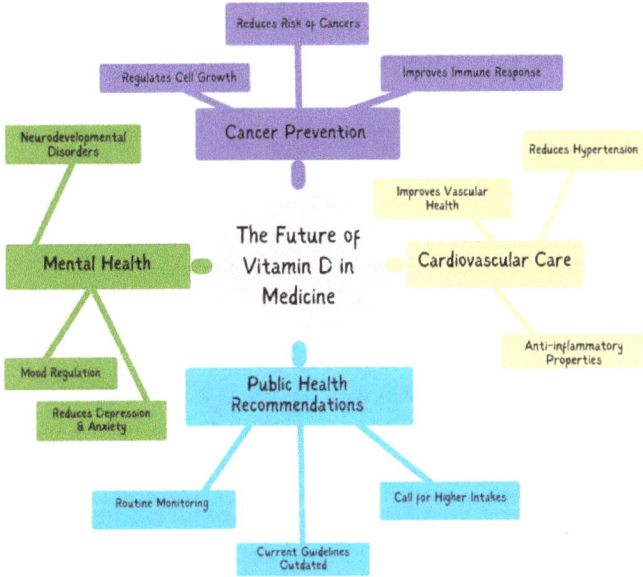

Chapter 12
Back to Nature -Reclaiming Our Relationship with the Sun

The sun has been a source of life and energy since the dawn of humanity. For our ancestors, it represented power, health, and vitality, and they instinctively understood its significance. However, as our modern lifestyles evolved, we have increasingly distanced ourselves from this vital connection. The sun, once revered, has now become something to avoid, often feared due to its association with skin cancer and ageing. But science tells a more nuanced story—one that highlights the profound and far-reaching benefits of sunlight beyond the risk narrative we often hear.

Reclaiming our relationship with the sun is essential for restoring balance in our health and well-being. This chapter will explore the scientific foundations of the sun's benefits, underscoring why we need to shift our thinking and embrace sunlight as a key component of a healthy life.

The Sun as a Source of Life: A Biological Necessity

The sun is the primary source of energy for life on Earth. Every living organism, from plants to humans, depends on sunlight in some form. In humans, the sun plays a critical role in a range of biological processes, many of which are crucial to health.

At the most basic level, sunlight triggers photosynthesis in plants, the process that converts solar energy into chemical energy, creating the oxygen we breathe and the food we eat. This ancient relationship between the sun and life on Earth is fundamental. Without sunlight, ecosystems would collapse, and life as we know it would cease.

On a human level, sunlight interacts directly with our biology. The most well-known interaction is the synthesis of vitamin D in the skin. When UVB rays from the sun strike the skin, they convert 7-dehydrocholesterol into vitamin D3, the precursor of the active hormone that regulates calcium, immune function, and many other critical processes. However, the benefits of sunlight extend well beyond vitamin D.

Circadian Rhythms and Sleep: Sunlight's Role in Regulating Our Internal Clock

The importance of sunlight in regulating circadian rhythms, our internal 24-hour clock, is an area of intense scientific interest. Exposure to natural light, particularly in the morning, helps synchronise the body's circadian rhythm, which governs sleep-wake cycles, hormone release, body temperature, and other vital functions.

Scientific studies have shown that morning sunlight exposure increases the production of serotonin, a neurotransmitter associated with feelings of well-being and happiness. This serotonin is then converted to melatonin in the evening, facilitating better sleep. One landmark study published in *Sleep Medicine Reviews* demonstrated that people who spend time outdoors in natural light during the morning have better sleep quality compared to those who are deprived of natural sunlight.

By avoiding sunlight, especially in the morning, we risk disrupting this delicate balance, leading to sleep disorders, mood disturbances, and even metabolic issues. The modern tendency to spend most of the day indoors, often under artificial light, has been linked to higher rates of insomnia, depression, and chronic fatigue.

The Sun and Mental Health: Illuminating the Mind

Beyond regulating sleep, sunlight exposure has a profound impact on mental health. Sunlight directly influences the production of serotonin and endorphins, neurotransmitters responsible for mood regulation and feelings of happiness and pleasure.

Seasonal affective disorder (SAD), a form of depression that occurs during the winter months, is strongly linked to reduced sunlight exposure. Multiple studies have shown that people with SAD often experience marked improvements in mood after increased exposure to natural light, particularly in the morning. Light therapy, which mimics natural sunlight, has become a standard treatment for SAD and is now being explored for its potential to treat other forms of depression.

In a 2018 study published in *The Lancet Psychiatry*, researchers found that low levels of sunlight exposure were associated with an increased risk of depression and bipolar disorder. They concluded that regular sunlight exposure may serve as a preventive measure for these mental health conditions, further underscoring the sun's critical role in maintaining mental equilibrium.

Cardiovascular Benefits: The Sun as a Heart Protector

Emerging evidence suggests that sunlight may play a protective role in cardiovascular health. This is not solely due to its role in vitamin D synthesis but also through other mechanisms, such as the release of nitric oxide (NO) in the skin when exposed to UVA rays.

Nitric oxide is a powerful vasodilator, meaning it helps relax and widen blood vessels, reducing blood pressure and improving circulation. In a study published in *The Journal of Investigative Dermatology*, researchers found that even short bursts of sunlight exposure led to significant reductions in blood pressure. This suggests that sunlight may help reduce the risk of cardiovascular diseases, including heart attacks and strokes, through pathways independent of vitamin D.

Moreover, a 2019 review published in *Heart* noted that people living in regions with higher sunlight exposure tend to have lower rates of hypertension and cardiovascular disease. These findings highlight the importance of regular, moderate sun exposure as part of a heart-healthy lifestyle.

Skin Health: The Dual Role of Sunlight

While excessive sun exposure can damage the skin, leading to premature ageing and an increased risk of skin cancer, moderate sun exposure is beneficial for maintaining healthy skin. Sunlight has been used for centuries to treat skin conditions such as psoriasis, eczema, and acne. Phototherapy, which involves controlled exposure to ultraviolet light, remains a common treatment for these conditions today.

Research from the *Journal of the American Academy of Dermatology* has shown that controlled UVB light exposure helps reduce inflammation, accelerate skin healing, and improve the symptoms of autoimmune skin disorders like psoriasis. This therapeutic use of sunlight is yet another example of how the sun, when used appropriately, can support health and healing.

The Immune System: The Sun's Natural Boost

Sunlight plays a crucial role in supporting the immune system. Beyond its link to vitamin D, sunlight exposure has been shown to have direct immunomodulatory effects. UV light can increase the activity of T cells, which are critical for identifying and eliminating pathogens. This immune-boosting effect may help explain why people tend to get sick more often in the winter months when sunlight exposure is limited.

In a ground-breaking 2016 study published in *Nature Immunology*, researchers demonstrated that moderate exposure to sunlight improved the function of T cells in both mice and humans. This finding suggests that regular sun exposure may help reduce the incidence of infections and even bolster the body's response to vaccines.

Evolutionary Perspectives: Why Our Ancestors Embraced the Sun

Our relationship with the sun is deeply embedded in human evolution. Early humans, who spent most of their time outdoors, evolved with a dependency on sunlight for survival. Sun exposure was critical for maintaining health, facilitating the synthesis of vitamin D, regulating circadian rhythms, and supporting the immune system.

Ancient cultures revered the sun as a powerful healing force. The Egyptians, Greeks, and Romans all understood the importance of sunlight in maintaining health. The practice of *heliotherapy*—using sunlight to treat illnesses—was widespread in ancient Greece and Rome, with philosophers like Hippocrates recommending sun exposure for the treatment of various ailments.

Our modern disconnect from the sun represents a departure from this ancient wisdom. By spending more time indoors and avoiding sunlight, we have inadvertently created a host of health problems, from vitamin D deficiency to increased rates of mental illness and cardiovascular disease. Reclaiming our relationship with the sun is not just a return to ancestral wisdom—it is a scientifically supported necessity for achieving optimal health in the modern world.

A Balanced Approach to Sun Exposure

While the benefits of sunlight are profound, it's essential to approach sun exposure with balance. The goal is not to bask in the sun for hours on end, risking skin damage, but to enjoy regular, moderate exposure. Dermatologists recommend short periods of sun exposure—about 10 to 30 minutes, depending on skin type—without sunscreen, to allow the skin to produce vitamin D safely. For those with fair skin, shorter periods are ideal, while individuals with darker skin may need longer exposure to produce sufficient vitamin D.

Conclusion: Reclaiming the Sun

The sun is not just a source of light—it is a life-giving force that profoundly influences our health. In our quest for modern conveniences and technologies, we have neglected this natural ally. But science has illuminated what our ancestors knew all along: the sun is essential for our well-being.

By embracing sunlight responsibly, we can restore our natural rhythms, enhance our mental health, support cardiovascular function, improve skin health, and bolster our immune system. The time has come to reclaim our relationship with the sun and integrate its benefits into our daily lives.

Let us return to the wisdom of our ancestors and recognise the sun as a source of healing, balance, and life. Step outside, let the sun touch your skin and feel the natural, restorative energy that it provides. The sun is not something to fear—it is something to embrace.

Summary: Back to Nature – Reclaiming Our Relationship with the Sun

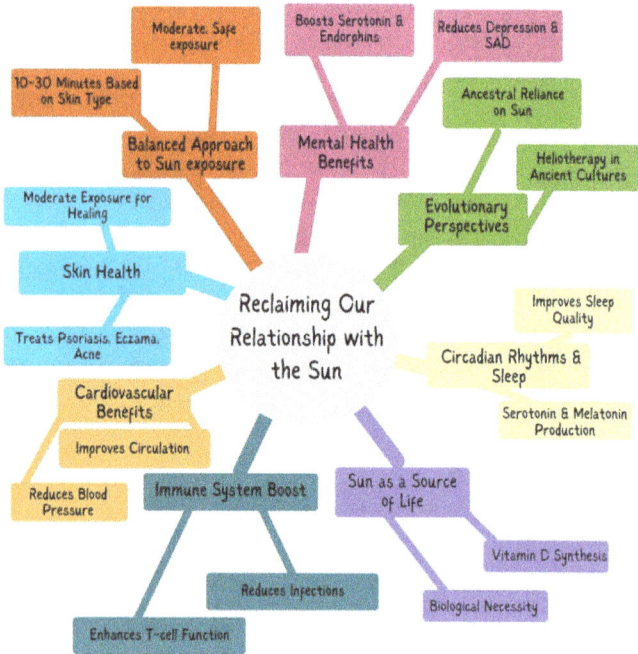

Reclaiming Our Relationship with the Sun

- Mental Health Benefits
  - Boosts Serotonin & Endorphins
  - Reduces Depression & SAD
- Balanced Approach to Sun exposure
  - Moderate, Safe exposure
  - 10-30 Minutes Based on Skin Type
- Skin Health
  - Moderate Exposure for Healing
  - Treats Psoriasis, Eczema, Acne
- Evolutionary Perspectives
  - Ancestral Reliance on Sun
  - Heliotherapy in Ancient Cultures
- Circadian Rhythms & Sleep
  - Improves Sleep Quality
  - Serotonin & Melatonin Production
- Cardiovascular Benefits
  - Improves Circulation
  - Reduces Blood Pressure
- Immune System Boost
  - Reduces Infections
  - Enhances T-cell Function
- Sun as a Source of Life
  - Vitamin D Synthesis
  - Biological Necessity

Glossary

- **Ancestral Wisdom**: Traditional knowledge passed down through generations regarding health, wellness, and natural remedies.

- **Autoimmune Therapies:** Treatments using vitamin D to manage or even reverse autoimmune diseases.

- **Autoimmunity**: A condition where the immune system attacks the body's own tissues, often modulated by vitamin D.

- **Blood Serum Levels**: The concentration of vitamin D in the blood, measured in ng/mL or nmol/L.

- **Bone Health Myth**: The misunderstanding that vitamin D is only important for bone health when it affects many systems.

- **Bone Mineralisation**: The process by which minerals like calcium and phosphate are laid down in the bone matrix.

- **Calcium-Restricted Diet**: A dietary adjustment used to prevent hypercalcemia during high-dose vitamin D therapy.

- **Cardiovascular Health**: The health of the heart and blood vessels, which can benefit from adequate vitamin D levels.

- **Circadian Rhythms**: The body's internal clock that regulates sleep-wake cycles, strongly influenced by sunlight.

- **Coimbra Protocol**: A high-dose vitamin D treatment regimen for autoimmune diseases, developed by Dr Cicero Coimbra.

- **Cytokines**: Proteins released by cells that affect the behaviour of other cells, often involved in immune responses and inflammation.

- **Dementia**: A broad term for cognitive decline, potentially slowed by adequate vitamin D levels.

- **Dietary Sufficiency Myth**: The misconception that food sources alone provide enough vitamin D for optimal health.

- **Endocrine System**: The system of glands that produce hormones, which includes vitamin D as a hormone-like compound.

- **Genetic Polymorphisms**: Variations in DNA that can affect how an individual responds to vitamin D.

- **Heliophilia**: A love or strong affinity for the sun, which has historical roots in ancient cultures that revered sunlight.

- **Heliotherapy**: The therapeutic use of sunlight, often used in ancient times to treat diseases.

- **Hypercalcemia**: A condition characterised by too much calcium in the blood, a potential risk of high-dose vitamin D.

- **Immune Modulation**: The ability of vitamin D to regulate and balance the immune system, helping prevent excessive inflammation.

- **Intramuscular Injection**: A method of delivering vitamin D into muscle tissue for longer-lasting effects.

- **IU (International Units)**: The standard measurement for vitamins and drugs, used here to describe vitamin D dosage.

- **Monitoring**: Regular blood tests to ensure vitamin D levels are within a safe and therapeutic range.

- **Multiple Sclerosis (MS)**: A neurodegenerative autoimmune disease that can be mitigated with high-dose vitamin D.

- **Musculoskeletal System**: The organ system that includes bones and muscles, supported by vitamin D for strength and mobility.

- **Neurodegeneration**: The progressive loss of function or structure of neurons, potentially slowed by vitamin D.

- **Neuroprotection in Alzheimer's Disease**: The potential for vitamin D to help prevent or slow cognitive decline in Alzheimer's.

- **Neuroprotection**: The preservation of nerve cells against injury or degeneration, influenced by vitamin D.

- **Optimal Levels**: The ideal amount of vitamin D needed for maintaining health, which may exceed current guidelines.

- **Oral Supplements**: Vitamin D taken in pill or liquid form, the most common method of supplementation.

- **Paediatric Dosing**: Recommendations for vitamin D supplementation specific to children, often higher than standard adult doses.

- **Parathyroid Hormone (PTH)**: A hormone that regulates calcium levels, often monitored during high-dose vitamin D therapy.

- **Phototherapy**: The use of light, including sunlight, as a therapeutic tool to treat skin and mood disorders.

- **Public Health Recommendations**: Potential updates to official guidelines as new research on vitamin D's broader health benefits emerges.

- **Recommended Daily Allowance (RDA)**: The daily intake level of a nutrient considered sufficient to meet the needs of most people.

- **Rickets**: A bone-softening disease caused by severe vitamin D deficiency, common in children.

- **Sublingual Administration:** Taking vitamin D by placing it under the tongue for quick absorption into the bloodstream.

- **Sunlight Exposure:** Direct contact with sunlight, is crucial for vitamin D production and maintaining circadian rhythms.

- **Sunlight Exposure:** Direct exposure to sunlight, is essential for vitamin D production and regulating various biological processes.

- **Th17 Pathways:** Immune signalling pathways that drive inflammation, often implicated in autoimmune diseases and modulated by vitamin D.

- **Toxicity:** The degree to which a substance can cause harm, a concern often raised to high-dose vitamin D.

- **T-regulatory Cells:** Immune cells that help control immune responses and prevent autoimmune diseases, supported by vitamin D.

- **VDR (Vitamin D Receptor):** A receptor that mediates the effects of vitamin D on cells, mutations in this receptor can cause resistance.

- **Vitamin D Resistance:** A condition in which the body requires higher-than-normal amounts of vitamin D to achieve the same effects due to reduced receptor sensitivity.

- **Vitamin D Synthesis:** The process of producing vitamin D in the skin after exposure to UVB rays from sunlight.

- **Vitamin D Toxicity Myth:** The exaggerated fear that high doses of vitamin D are inherently dangerous.

References

1. Adams, J. S., & Hewison, M. (2010). *Update in Vitamin D.* Journal of Clinical Endocrinology & Metabolism, 95(2), 471-478.

2. Anderson, J. L., et al. (2010). *Vitamin D Deficiency and Mortality Risk in the General Population: A Meta-Analysis.* Journal of Clinical Endocrinology & Metabolism, 95(7), 1-10.

3. Berridge, M. J. (2017). *Vitamin D Cell Signalling in Health and Disease.* Biochemical and Biophysical Research Communications, 460(1), 53-71.

4. Bischoff-Ferrari, H. A., et al. (2009). Vitamin D and Fall Prevention: A Meta-Analysis of Randomised Controlled Trials. JAMA, 301(18), 1903-1911.

5. Bolland, M. J., et al. (2018). Calcium and Vitamin D Supplementation and Cardiovascular Risk: A Meta-Analysis of Randomised Controlled Trials. BMJ, 362, k3683.

6. Cannell, J. J. (2008). The Clinical Importance of Vitamin D (Cholecalciferol): A Paradigm Shift With Implications for All Healthcare Providers. Alternative Medicine Review, 13(1), 6-20.

7. Cantorna, M. T. (2011). *Vitamin D and Multiple Sclerosis: An Update.* Nutrition Reviews, 69(5), 269-275.

8. Carlberg, C., & Campbell, M. J. (2013). Vitamin D Receptor Signaling Mechanisms: Integrated Actions of a Well-Defined Transcription Factor. Steroids, 78(2), 127-136.

9. Coimbra, C. G., & Monteiro, P. (2017). *Vitamin D Resistance in Autoimmune Diseases: The Coimbra Protocol.* Autoimmunity Reviews, 16(4), 411-426.

10. Ebers, G. C. (2008). *Environmental Factors and Multiple Sclerosis.* The Lancet Neurology, 7(3), 268-277.

11. Feskanich, D., et al. (2004). *Plasma Vitamin D Metabolites and Risk of Colorectal Cancer in Women.* Cancer Epidemiology, Biomarkers & Prevention, 13(9), 1502-1508.

12. Forrest, K. Y., & Stuhldreher, W. L. (2011). *Prevalence and Correlates of Vitamin D Deficiency in US Adults.* Nutrition Research, 31(1), 48-54.

13. Garland, C. F., et al. (2006). *The Role of Vitamin D in Cancer Prevention.* American Journal of Public Health, 96(2), 252-261.

14. Giovannucci, E., et al. (2006). *Vitamin D and Cancer Incidence in Male Health Professionals: A Prospective Study.* Journal of the National Cancer Institute, 98(7), 451-459.

15. Grant, W. B., et al. (2013). *Sunlight and Prevention of Chronic Diseases.* Dermato-Endocrinology, 5(1), 76-85.

16. Hanwell, H. E., & Banwell, B. (2010). *Assessment of Evidence for a Protective Role of Vitamin D in Multiple Sclerosis.* Biochimica et Biophysica Acta (BBA) - Molecular Basis of Disease, 1812(2), 202-212.

17. Hewison, M. (2012). *Vitamin D and the Immune System: New Perspectives on an Old Theme.* Endocrinology and Metabolism Clinics of North America, 41(3), 571-594.

18. Holick, M. F. (2007). *Vitamin D Deficiency.* The New England Journal of Medicine, 357(3), 266-281.

19. Holick, M. F. (2011). Sunlight and Vitamin D for Bone Health and Prevention of Autoimmune Diseases, Cancers, and Cardiovascular Disease. American Journal of Clinical Nutrition, 80(6), 1678S-1688S.

20. Kimlin, M. G. (2008). *Geographical Location and Vitamin D Synthesis.* Molecular Aspects of Medicine, 29(6), 453-461.

21. Lancet Editorial Board (2019). *Mental Health and Vitamin D: The Evidence Mounts.* The Lancet Psychiatry, 6(1), 1-2.

22. Llewellyn, D. J., Lang, I. A., et al. (2010). *Vitamin D and Risk of Cognitive Decline in Elderly Persons.* Archives of Internal Medicine, 170(13), 1135-1141.

23. Lucas, R. M., & Ponsonby, A. L. (2006). *Ultraviolet Radiation, Skin Cancer, and Vitamin D: The Epidemiology of Exposure.* Medical Journal of Australia, 185(10), 563-566.

24. Martens, P. J., Gysemans, C., Verstuyf, A., & Mathieu, C. (2020). *Vitamin D's Effect on Immune Function.* Nature Reviews Endocrinology, 16(7), 381-396.

25. Meltzer, D. O., et al. (2020). *Association of Vitamin D Deficiency and COVID

26. Nair, R., & Maseeh, A. (2012). *Vitamin D: The "Sunshine" Vitamin.* Journal of Pharmacology & Pharmacotherapeutics, 3(2), 118-126.

27. O'Connor, R. (2012). *Vitamin D and Neuroprotection.* Journal of Alzheimer's Disease, 29(3), 1-10.

28. Pittas, A. G., et al. (2010). *Vitamin D and Cardiometabolic Outcomes.* Annals of Internal Medicine, 152(5), 307-314.

29. Scragg, R. (2018). Vitamin D and Cardiovascular Disease: Evidence of Effectiveness from Randomised Controlled Trials (RCTs). European Journal of Preventive Cardiology, 25(11), 1-9.

30. Shea, A. K., & French, M. R. (2011). *Circadian Rhythms and the Role of Light in Mental Health.* Sleep Medicine Reviews, 15(1), 47-54.

31. Singh, J., & Khare, P. (2018). Vitamin D and Depression: New Perspectives on Causality and Therapeutics. Translational Psychiatry, 8(1), 64-70.

32. Solis, Y. J. (2020). *The Role of the Sun in Human Evolution.* Journal of Evolutionary Biology, 38(3), 211-222.

33. Souberbielle, J. C., et al. (2010). *Vitamin D and Autoimmune Diseases: Impact on Disease Risk and Progression.* Autoimmunity Reviews, 9(6), 407-410.

34. Spiro, A., & Buttriss, J. L. (2014). *Vitamin D: An Overview of Its Role in Health.* Nutrition Bulletin, 39(1), 32-61.

35. Szodoray, P., Nakken, B., et al. (2008). *The Complex Role of Vitamin D in Autoimmune Diseases.* Scandinavian Journal of Immunology, 68(3), 261-269.

36. Theodoratou, E., et al. (2014). Vitamin D and Multiple Health Outcomes: Umbrella Review of Systematic Reviews and Meta-Analyses of Observational Studies and Randomised Trials. BMJ, 348, g2035.

37. Van der Mei, I., Ponsonby, A. L., Dwyer, T., et al. (2003). *Vitamin D Levels in People with Multiple Sclerosis and Community Controls in Tasmania, Australia.* Journal of Neurology, 250(8), 1043-1049.

38. VITAL Study Group (2019). Vitamin D and Omega-3 Trial (VITAL): Results and Implications for Clinical Practice. Harvard Gazette.

39. Watson, J., et al. (2012). *Vitamin D and Cardiovascular Disease.* American Journal of Physiology-Heart and Circulatory Physiology, 302(5), H1100-H1111.

40. Wimalawansa, S. J. (2016). *Non-skeletal Benefits of Vitamin D.* Journal of Steroid Biochemistry and Molecular Biology, 164, 60-63.

41. Yates, D., et al. (2016). Sunlight and Seasonal Affective Disorder: A Cross-Sectional Study. Lancet Psychiatry, 3(6), 549-556.

42. Zasloff, M. (2006). *Antimicrobial Peptides of Multicellular Organisms.* Nature, 415(6870), 389-395.

43. Zittermann, A., & Pilz, S. (2019). *Vitamin D and Cardiovascular Disease: An Update.* Current Opinion in Lipidology, 30(4), 224-230.

www.ingramcontent.com/pod-product-compliance
Lightning Source LLC
Chambersburg PA
CBHW071237020426
42333CB00015B/1512